T0226404

Autism Spectrum Disorder across the Lifespan Part II

Editors

ROBERT W. WISNER-CARLSON
SCOTT R. PEKRUL
THOMAS FLIS
ROBERT SCHLOESSER

PSYCHIATRIC CLINICS
OF NORTH AMERICA

www.psych.theclinics.com

Consulting Editor
HARSH K. TRIVEDI

March 2021 • Volume 44 • Number 1

ELSEVIER

1600 John F. Kennedy Boulevard • Suite 1800 • Philadelphia, Pennsylvania, 19103-2899

http://www.theclinics.com

PSYCHIATRIC CLINICS OF NORTH AMERICA Volume 44, Number 1
March 2021 ISSN 0193-953X, ISBN-13: 978-0-323-83608-1

Editor: Lauren Boyle
Developmental Editor: Nicole Congleton

Psychiatric Clinics of North America (ISSN 0193-953X) is published quarterly by Elsevier Inc., 360 Park Avenue South, New York, NY 10010-1710. Months of issue are March, June, September, and December. Business and Editorial Offices: 1600 John F. Kennedy Blvd., Suite 1800, Philadelphia, PA 19103-2899. Periodicals postage paid at New York, NY and additional mailing offices. Subscription prices are $338.00 per year (US individuals), $966.00 per year (US institutions), $100.00 per year (US students/residents), $406.00 per year (Canadian individuals), $499.00 per year (international individuals), $1024.00 per year (Canadian & international institutions), and $220.00 per year (international students/residents), $100.00 per year (Canadian & students/residents). Foreign air speed delivery is included in all *Clinics'* subscription prices. All prices are subject to change without notice. **POSTMASTER:** Send address changes to *Psychiatric Clinics of North America*, Elsevier Health Sciences Division, Subscription Customer Service, 3251 Riverport Lane, Maryland Heights, MO 63043. **Customer Service: 1-800-654-2452 (US). From outside the United States, call 1-314-447-8871. Fax: 1-314-447-8029. E-mail: journalscustomerservice-usa@elsevier.com (for print support) and journalsonlinesupport-usa@elsevier.com (for online support).**

Reprints. For copies of 100 or more, of articles in this publication, please contact the Commercial Reprints Department, Elsevier Inc., 360 Park Avenue South, New York, New York 10010-1710. Tel.: 212-633-3874, Fax: 212-633-3820, E-mail: reprints@elsevier.com.

Psychiatric Clinics of North America is covered in *MEDLINE/PubMed (Index Medicus), Current Contents/Social and Behavioral Sciences, Social Science Citation Index, Embase/Excerpta Medica,* and PsycINFO.

Contributors

CONSULTING EDITOR

HARSH K. TRIVEDI, MD, MBA
President and Chief Executive Officer, Sheppard Pratt Health System, Baltimore, Maryland, USA

EDITORS

ROBERT W. WISNER-CARLSON, MD
Medical Director, Neuropsychiatry Outpatient Program, Director, Adult Developmental Neuropsychiatry Clinic, Senior Psychiatrist and Service Chief, Adult Inpatient Intellectual Disability and Autism Unit, Clinician Investigator, Sheppard Pratt Autism Registry, Chairman, Ethics Committee, Sheppard Pratt Hospital, Adjunct Assistant Professor, University of Maryland School of Medicine, Baltimore, Maryland, USA

SCOTT R. PEKRUL, MD
Service Chief, Child and Adolescent Inpatient Neuropsychiatric Unit, Sheppard Pratt Health System, Baltimore, Maryland, USA

THOMAS FLIS, MS, BCBA, LBA, LCPC
Behavioral Services Manager, Sheppard Pratt Health System, Baltimore, Maryland, USA

ROBERT SCHLOESSER, MD
Director, Point-of-Care Research and Innovation, Associate Chief Medical Information Officer, Sheppard Pratt Health System, Baltimore, Maryland, USA

AUTHORS

LAURA ANDERSEN, MD
Clinical Instructor, Department of Psychiatry, University of Michigan, University of Michigan Medical Center, Ann Arbor, Michigan, USA

KELLY B. BECK, PhD
Assistant Professor, Department of Rehabilitation Science and Technology, University of Pittsburgh School of Health and Rehabilitation Sciences, Pittsburgh, Pennsylvania, USA

FRANK M.C. BESAG, ChB, FRCP, FRCPsych, FRCPCH
Professor, East London NHS Foundation Trust, Bedford, United Kingdom; University College London, King's College London, London, United Kingdom

KAITLYN E. BREITENFELDT, BS
Research Assistant, Department of Psychiatry, University of Pittsburgh School of Medicine, Pittsburgh, Pennsylvania, USA

CAITLIN M. CONNER, PhD
Research Assistant Professor, Department of Psychiatry, University of Pittsburgh School of Medicine, Pittsburgh, Pennsylvania, USA

JENNIFER LOUISE COOK, PhD (Neuroscience)
Senior Research Fellow, School of Psychology, University of Birmingham, Birmingham, United Kingdom

MOHAMMAD GHAZIUDDIN, MD
Professor of Psychiatry, University of Michigan, University of Michigan Medical Center, Ann Arbor, Michigan, USA

NEERA GHAZIUDDIN, MD, MRCPsych(UK)
Professor of Psychiatry, University of Michigan, University of Michigan Medical Center, Ann Arbor, Michigan, USA

MARCO GRADOS, MD, MPH
Johns Hopkins School of Medicine, Baltimore, Maryland, USA

MERRILYN HOOLEY, PhD
Senior Lecturer, Department of Psychology, Deakin University, Geelong, Victoria, Australia

SANJAY KAJI, MD
Johns Hopkins Hospital, Baltimore, Maryland, USA

CONNOR TOM KEATING, Psychology BSc (Hons)
PhD Student, School of Psychology, University of Birmingham, Birmingham, United Kingdom

ELIZABETH KUNREUTHER, MSW, LCSW, LCAS
Clinical Instructor, Department of Psychiatry, UNC School of Medicine, Chapel Hill, North Carolina, USA

MONEEK MADRA, PhD
Department of Pediatrics, Morgan Stanley Children's Hospital, Institute of Human Nutrition, Columbia University Irving Medical Center, New York, New York, USA

KARA GROSS MARGOLIS, MD
Department of Pediatrics, Morgan Stanley Children's Hospital, Institute of Human Nutrition, Columbia University Irving Medical Center, New York, New York, USA

CARLA A. MAZEFSKY, PhD
Associate Professor, Department of Psychiatry, University of Pittsburgh School of Medicine, Pittsburgh, Pennsylvania, USA

GARY B. MESIBOV, PhD
Professor Emeritus, Division TEACCH, UNC School of Medicine, University of North Carolina, Chapel Hill, North Carolina, USA

JESSIE B. NORTHRUP, PhD
Postdoctoral Fellow, Department of Psychiatry, University of Pittsburgh School of Medicine, Pittsburgh, Pennsylvania, USA

SA EUN PARK, MD
Kennedy Krieger Institute, Baltimore, Maryland, USA

LAURA A. PECORA, BA, PGDip(Psych)
Research Student, Department of Psychology, Deakin University, Geelong, Victoria, Australia

ROEY RINGEL
Department of Pediatrics, Morgan Stanley Children's Hospital, Columbia University Irving Medical Center, Columbia College, Columbia University, New York, New York, USA

BENJAMIN SARCIA, MA, BCBA, LBA
Program Director, Healthy Beginnings Feeding Therapy Program, Verbal Beginnings, LLC, Columbia, Maryland, USA

LAURIE SPERRY, PhD, BCBA-D
Adjunct Lecturer, Department of Psychiatry and Behavioral Sciences, Division of General Psychiatry and Psychology, School of Medicine, Stanford University, Stanford, California, USA

MARK A. STOKES, PhD
Associate Professor, Department of Psychology, Deakin University, Geelong, Victoria, Australia

MICHAEL J. VASEY, BSc
Research Assistant to Frank M.C. Besag, East London NHS Foundation Trust, Bedford, United Kingdom

LEE WACHTEL, MD
Johns Hopkins School of Medicine, Kennedy Krieger Institute, Baltimore, Maryland, USA

SUSAN W. WHITE, PhD
Doddridge Franklin Saxon Endowed Chair in Clinical Psychology, Director of Center for the Prevention of Youth Behavior Problems, Center for Youth Development and Intervention, Department of Psychology, University of Alabama, Tuscaloosa, Alabama, USA

Contents

Autism seldom occurs in its pure form. Often labeled as behavioral disorders or psychological reactions, comorbid psychiatric disorders are common. Bipolar disorder is one of the most common psychiatric disorders that occur in persons with autism across their life spans. It can be comorbid with and mistaken for several other conditions. Similarly, psychosis occurs in several psychiatric disorders. Schizophrenia is the prototype psychotic disorder that has a close but controversial relationship with autism. Assessment and treatment of bipolar disorder and psychosis should be based on their individual characteristics, family dynamics, and community resources.

 Video content accompanies this article at http://www.childpsych. theclinics.com.

Catatonia was first described by Karl Ludwig Kahlbaum in 1874, occurring in association with other psychiatric and medical disorders. However, in the nineteenth century the disorder was incorrectly classified as a subtype of schizophrenia. This misclassification persisted until the publication of DSM-5 in 2013 when important changes were incorporated. Although the etiology is unknown, disrupted gamma-aminobutyric acid has been proposed as the underlying pathophysiological mechanism. Key symptoms can be identified under 3 clinical domains: motor, speech, and behavioral. Benzodiazepines and electroconvulsive therapy are the only known effective treatments. Timely recognition and treatment have important outcome, and sometimes lifesaving, implications.

The mechanism of action of electroconvulsive therapy (ECT) is not fully elucidated, with prevailing theories ranging from neuroendocrinological to neuroplasticity effects of ECT or epileptiform brain plasticity. Youth with autism can present with catatonia. ECT is a treatment that can safely and rapidly resolve catatonia in autism and should be considered promptly. The literature available for ECT use in youth with autism is consistently growing. Under-recognition of the catatonic syndrome and delayed diagnosis and implementation of the anticatatonic treatment paradigms, including ECT, as well as stigma and lack of knowledge of ECT remain clinical stumbling blocks.

Kelly B. Beck, Caitlin M. Conner, Kaitlyn E. Breitenfeldt, Jessie B. Northrup, Susan W. White, and Carla A. Mazefsky

Emotion regulation (ER) is the ability to modify arousal and emotional reactivity to achieve goals and maintain adaptive behaviors. ER impairment in autism spectrum disorder (ASD) is thought to underlie many problem behaviors, co-occurring psychiatric symptoms, and social impairment, and yet is largely unaddressed both clinically and in research. There is a critical need to develop ER treatment and assessment options for individuals with ASD across the life span, given the multitude of downstream effects on functioning. This article summarizes the current state of science in ER assessment and treatment and identifies the most promising measurement options and treatments.

Laura A. Pecora, Merrilyn Hooley, Laurie Sperry, Gary B. Mesibov, and Mark A. Stokes

This article reviews relevant literature on sexuality in individuals with autism spectrum disorder (ASD). Findings reveal a growing awareness of desire for sexual and intimate relationships in individuals with ASD. However, core impairments of ASD lead to difficulties establishing requisite knowledge and skills necessary to attain a healthy sexuality and facilitate relationships. Consequently, individuals with ASD present with increased risk of engaging in inappropriate sexual behaviors and sexual victimization than their typically developing peers. The literature asserts the need to implement effective sexual education programs to assist in development of healthy sexual identity and relationships that meet each individual's needs.

Connor Tom Keating and Jennifer Louise Cook

Social "difficulties" associated with ASD may be a product of neurotypical-autistic differences in emotion expression and recognition. Research suggests that neurotypical and autistic individuals exhibit expressive differences, with autistic individuals displaying less frequent expressions that are rated lower in quality by non-autistic raters. Autistic individuals have difficulties recognizing neurotypical facial expressions; neurotypical individuals have difficulties recognizing autistic expressions. However, findings are mixed. Task-related factors (e.g., intensity of stimuli) and participant characteristics (e.g., age, IQ, comorbid diagnoses) may contribute to the mixed findings. The authors conclude by highlighting important areas for future research and the clinical implications of the discussed findings.

PSYCHIATRIC CLINICS OF NORTH AMERICA

SERIES OF RELATED INTEREST

Child and Adolescent Psychiatric Clinics of North America
https://www.childpsych.theclinics.com/

Neurologic Clinics
https://www.neurologic.theclinics.com/

THE CLINICS ARE AVAILABLE ONLINE!
Access your subscription at:
www.theclinics.com

Preface

Acts of Medical Kindness for People with Autism

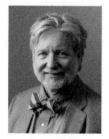 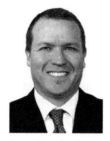 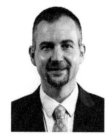

Robert W. Wisner-Carlson, MD   Scott R. Pekrul, MD   Thomas Flis, MS, BCBA, LBA, LCPC

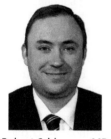

Robert Schloesser, MD

Editors

April 2020 began a "Year of Kindness" for people with autism spectrum disorder (ASD), with a call for "one million acts of kindness, big and small."[1] Acts of kindness are needed more than ever for everyone, particularly our patients with ASD, amid the increased anxiety, uncertainty, and even terror inflicted by a pandemic that has dramatically altered daily routines and mandated social distancing. For physicians and other mental health clinicians, medical acts of kindness must be underpinned by professional knowledge and humanizing clinical experiences for this growing patient population. Recently released Centers for Disease Control and Prevention data reveal the increased prevalence of ASD in 8-year-olds across the United States: one in 54 (18.5 per 1000)[2] in 2016, compared with one in 59 in the last reporting period (2014).[3] With the prevalence of ASD now approaching 2%, the relevant body of medical knowledge must include an appreciation of the various burdens associated with this neurodevelopmental disorder beyond impairments in social cognition and communication. For this reason, psychiatric and medical comorbidities are the focus of the second issue in this 2-part series.

Psychiatr Clin N Am 44 (2021) xi–xiv
https://doi.org/10.1016/j.psc.2021.01.001
0193-953X/21/© 2021 Published by Elsevier Inc.

psych.theclinics.com

Psychiatric and medical comorbidities occur at increased rates in individuals with ASD.[4–7] Obsessive compulsive disorder and the intersection of eating disorders and the female profile of ASD were reviewed in Part I. In Part II, additional psychiatric conditions are considered. Ghaziuddin and Ghaziuddin review the comorbidity of ASD with bipolar disorder and psychosis. As well, Ghaziuddin, Andersen, and Ghaziuddin review catatonia in ASD, a condition increasingly recognized as cooccurring and sometimes requiring life-saving treatment. Electroconvulsive therapy can be that life-saving treatment, and its use in ASD comorbidities is reviewed by Park, Grados, Wachtel, and Kaji. Substance use disorders have been thought to be less prevalent in people with ASD compared with the general population. Kenreuther questions this assumption and explores how constructed narratives can bias us as clinicians treating the ASD population.

Medical comorbidities also are prevalent, and 2 common ones are considered in this issue. Besag and Vasey review seizures and epilepsy in ASD, an association which turns out to be bidirectional. Gastrointestinal issues, a frequent problem and potential cause of behavioral dysregulation in autism, is reviewed by Madra, Ringel, and Margolis. Not all issues with food, though, are medical issues, per se. Sarcia reviews the types of dysfunctional meal-time behaviors requiring intervention with applied behavioral analysis. Emotional dysregulation is a common source of suffering for people with autism. The assessment and treatment of emotional regulation impairments is reviewed by Beck, Conner, Breitenfeldt, Northrup, White, and Mazefsky.

The psychiatric assessment of individuals with ASD requires a special approach and a degree of flexibility. Because of the increased prevalence of intellectual disability (ID)[2] and the concreteness of thought irrespective of IQ,[8–10] the clinician must take special care in the psychiatric interview and mental status examination. Collateral informants are almost always needed. One must be careful in the way one asks questions, taking care with metaphorical language and complex grammar. One must sometimes take a special approach to diagnosis, especially in those ASD patients with comorbid ID. Manuals such as the DM-ID-2 of the National Association of Dual Diagnoses[11] (the dual diagnoses being mental health disorders and developmental disabilities) and the DC-LD, an occasional paper of the Royal College of Psychiatrists in collaboration with the Penrose Society describing diagnostic criteria for psychiatric disorders for use with adults with learning disabilities/ID,[12] can assist the clinician in making psychiatric diagnoses in individuals with ASD. Common presenting problems, including aggression and self-injurious behaviors, are nonspecific and may relate to a medical condition causing pain or discomfort, such as dental pain, or to a psychiatric condition, or to an unexpected change in routine or environment. The clinician must carefully assess and investigate differential diagnoses. The approach described by McHugh and Slavney in *The Perspectives of Psychiatry* is applicable to this patient population as well.[13,14]

Other burdens arise for individuals on the autism spectrum. Sexuality and gender issues are reviewed by Pecora, Hooley, Sperry, Mesibov, and Stokes. The complexity of these issues, the normal desires, and the sometimes awkward approaches can complicate and befuddle the life of those with autism. Surprising to some clinicians may be the higher incidence of transgenderism in people with ASD, compared with the general population.

Finally, Keating and Cook return to the issue of how individuals with ASD differ from neurotypical individuals, in particular, in the production and interpretation of facial expressions. Understanding the phenomenal world of our patients is furthered by our ability to "put ourselves in their shoes." Keating and Cook help us to appreciate the neurotypical-autistic miscommunications that occur in this nonverbal way of interacting.

Therefore, in this 2-part series on ASD across the lifespan, numerous topics have been considered: from the initial diagnosis of ASD, to comorbid conditions, to the vagaries of traversing the phases and transitions of life. The prevalence of ASD in young people has increased by more than 250%[15] in the past 2 decades, either because of the heightened awareness of autism or because of other factors. Mental health professionals have much to offer individuals with autism at every stage of life. A thorough understanding of the psychiatric and medical burdens and barriers these individuals face and a commitment to address them in treatment will go a long way to achieving a million acts of kindness. Our patients with ASD, who sometimes seem to lack empathy, need it from us more than ever.

Robert W. Wisner-Carlson, MD
Sheppard Pratt Health System
6501 North Charles Street
Baltimore, MD 21204, USA

Scott R. Pekrul, MD
Sheppard Pratt Health System
6501 North Charles Street
Baltimore, MD 21204, USA

Thomas Flis, MS, BCBA, LBA, LCPC
Sheppard Pratt Health System
6501 North Charles Street
Baltimore, MD 21204, USA

Robert Schloesser, MD
Sheppard Pratt Health System
6501 North Charles Street
Baltimore, MD 21204, USA

E-mail addresses:
RWisner-Carlson@sheppardpratt.org (R.W. Wisner-Carlson)
SPekrul@sheppardpratt.org (S.R. Pekrul)
tflis@sheppardpratt.org (T. Flis)
rschloesser@sheppardpratt.org (R. Schloesser)

REFERENCES

1. World Autism Awareness Month FAQ. Available at: https://www.autismspeaks.org/world-autism-month-faq. Accessed March 29, 2020.

2. Maenner MJ, Shaw KA, Baio J, et al. Prevalence of autism spectrum disorder among children aged 8 years—autism and developmental disabilities monitoring network, 11 sites, United States, 2016. MMWR Surveill Summ 2020;69(4):1–12. https://doi.org/10.15585/mmwr.ss6904a1.

3. Baio J, Wiggins L, Christensen DL, et al. Prevalence of autism spectrum disorder among children aged 8 years–autism and developmental disabilities monitoring network, 11 sites, United States, 2014. MMWR Surveill Summ 2018;67(6):1–23. https://doi.org/10.15585/mmwr.ss6706a1.

4. Lai M-C, Kassee C, Besney R, et al. Prevalence of co-occurring mental health diagnoses in the autism population: a systematic review and meta-analysis. Lancet Psychiatry 2019;6:819–29. https://doi.org/10.1016/S2215-0366(19)30289-5.

5. Levy SE, Giarelli E, Lee LC, et al. Autism spectrum disorder and co-occurring developmental, psychiatric, and medical conditions among children in multiple populations of the United States. J Dev Behav Pediatr 2010;31:267–75. https://doi.org/10.1097/DBP.0b013e3181d5d03b.

6. Davignon MN, Qian Y, Massolo M, Croen LA. Psychiatric and medical conditions in transition-aged individuals with ASD. Pediatrics 2018;141(suppl 4):S335–45. https://doi.org/10.1542/peds.2016-4300K.

7. Kirsch AC, Huebner ARS, Mehta SQ, et al. Association of comorbid mood and anxiety disorders with autism spectrum disorder. JAMA Pediatr 2020;174(1):63–70. https://doi.org/10.1001/jamapediatrics.2019.4368.

8. Kalandadze T, Norbury C, Nærland T, et al. Figurative language comprehension in individuals with autism spectrum disorder: a meta-analytic review. Autism 2018;22(2):99–117.

9. Kanner L. Autistic disturbances of affective contact. Nerv Child 1943;2:217–50. https://doi.org/10.1111/fwb.12896.

10. Rumsey JM, Rapoport JL, Sceery WR. Autistic children as adults: psychiatric, social, and behavioral outcomes. J Am Acad Child Psychiatry 1985;24(4):465–73.

11. Fletcher RJ, Barnhill J, Cooper SA. DM-ID 2. Diagnostic manual—intellectual disability: a textbook of diagnosis of mental disorders in persons with intellectual disability. J Ment Health Res Intellect Disabil 2016;29.

12. Psychiatrists RC of, Group DDW DC-LD: diagnostic criteria for psychiatric disorders for use with adults with learning disabilities/mental retardation. Royal College of Psychiatrists Occasional Paper OP 48, London: Gaskell, 2001. p. 128.

13. McHugh PR, Slavney PR. The perspectives of psychiatry. Baltimore (MD): JHU Press; 1998.

14. Harris JC. Multimodal intervention for developmental neuropsychiatric disorders. In: Gillberg C, O'Brien G, editors. Clinics in Developmental Medicine No. 149: Developmental Disability and Behaviour. London: Mac Keith Press; 2000. p. 125–37.

15. Data and statistics on autism spectrum disorder. Centers for Disease Control and Prevention. Available at: https://www.cdc.gov/ncbddd/autism/data.html. Accessed March 29, 2020.

Bipolar Disorder and Psychosis in Autism

Mohammad Ghaziuddin, MD*, Neera Ghaziuddin, MD, MRCPsych(UK)

KEYWORDS

- Bipolar disorder • Psychosis • Autism • Asperger syndrome

KEY POINTS

- Bipolar disorder and psychosis are severe comorbid psychiatric disorders that can occur in persons with autism spectrum disorders (ASDs).
- Although classified as distinct conditions, they can occur together or at different times across the life span of a person with autism.
- Persons with ASD are probably at an increased risk of developing these conditions compared with the general population.
- Their diagnosis, treatments, and outcomes are complicated by the heterogeneity of ASD and by the co-occurrence of other medical and psychiatric disorders.

BIPOLAR DISORDER

In its classic form, bipolar disorder is one of the most severe psychiatric disorders that can co-occur in persons with autism spectrum disorders (ASDs). Along with depression and anxiety, it is probably the most common psychiatric disorder that occurs with autism. Before examining its comorbidity with autism, it is important to briefly review its current classification. The Diagnostic and Statistical Manual of Mental Disorders, Fifth Revision (DSM-5) classifies it as bipolar I, bipolar II, and cyclothymic disorders.[1] Bipolar I disorder represents classic manic-depressive disorder when a person has a manic episode, with or without depression or psychosis. Bipolar II disorder is diagnosed in the presence of at least 1 major depressive episode and at least 1 hypomanic episode by history. Patients return to their usual levels of functioning between the episodes. People with bipolar II often first seek treatment because of depressive symptoms, which can be severe. Cyclothymic disorder represents a milder form of bipolar disorder with a history of mood swings of at least 2 years' duration. The DSM-5 also has a residual category of other specified bipolar and related disorders

This article originally appeared in *Child and Adolescent Psychiatric Clinics*, Volume 29, Issue 3, July 2020.
University of Michigan, University of Michigan Medical Center, 4250 Plymouth Road, Ann Arbor, MI 48109, USA
* Corresponding author.
E-mail address: mghaziud@umich.edu

when the criteria for any of the 3 specific categories are not met. Bipolar disorder itself can be comorbid with and mistaken for several conditions, such as anxiety disorders, substance abuse, attention-deficit/hyperactivity disorder (ADHD), and oppositional defiant disorder not only in the general population but also in persons with ASDs.[2]

Prevalence

The exact prevalence of bipolar disorder in children with autism in the community is not clear. Some clinic-based studies have suggested high rates. For example, Worzniak and colleagues[3] found that 21% of an outpatient sample of children with ASD had bipolar disorder. Somewhat higher rates have been reported in some clinical studies of adults with ASD.[4] For example, in a study of 44 adult outpatients with ASD, Munesue and colleagues[5] reported that 16 (34%) had a mood disorder. Out of these, 4 were diagnosed with major depression, 2 with bipolar I, 6 with bipolar II, and 4 with bipolar disorder not otherwise specified. Thus, in all, 12 (75%) were diagnosed with some form of bipolar disorder.

Presentation

Both autism and bipolar disorder may present to medical attention with the symptoms of irritability and aggression. However, these are not the core symptoms of either disorder. Although reciprocal social and communicative deficits with restricted interests and behaviors form the core features of autism, mood symptoms, particularly grandiosity, are typical of bipolar disorder. When a person with autism presents with mood and behavior changes during episodes that represent a change from the patient's usual behavior, bipolar disorder should be ruled out. However, its presentation in autism may present unique challenges[6] depending on several factors, such as age, the subtype of bipolar disorder, the subtype of ASD, the presence of intellectual disability, and the presence of concurrent psychiatric and medical comorbidity. Sapmaz and colleagues[7] (2018) compared 40 children with ASD with bipolar disorder with a matched group of 40 children with ASD without bipolar disorder on several rating scales (Aberrant Behavior Checklist and the Young Mania Rating Scale–Parent Version). The former group showed a "highly episodic course, with manic episodes, subsyndromal symptoms and inter-episodic periods commonly being described in the manic symptom profile of these children."[7] This study included children with intellectual disability; however, the ASD plus bipolar group had more patients with ADHD than the ASD-only group. Joshi and colleagues[8] (2013) suggested that grandiosity was a dominant symptom in ASD symptoms with bipolar disorder. However, their study excluded patients with intellectual disability. In summary, classic bipolar disorder is most easily recognized in high-functioning verbal individuals with ASD by the presence of distinct alternating cycles of elated and depressed mood. The diagnostic confidence decreases with the intelligence quotient (IQ). In the low-functioning group, aggressive behavior, irritability, and hyperactivity may be more common during the hypomanic phases, whereas loss of weight and appetite, sleep disturbance, and decreased communication may be more common during the depressed phase. In addition, the symptoms may be modified by the presence of other medical and psychiatric comorbidities.

Cause

It is likely that the same factors that contribute to the cause of bipolar disorder in the general population also play a role in its comorbidity with autism. Studies have suggested that the risk of depression, including possibly bipolar disorder, is increased in the parents of autistic children. Genetic studies have identified common genes for autism, schizophrenia, and bipolar disorder, among others.[9,10]

Complications

Increased morbidity
Having both autism and bipolar disorder increases the functional impairment of the patient and the burden of care of the family.[11]

Suicidal risk
Suicidal risk can be divided into suicidal ideation, suicidal behavior, and completed suicide. In clinical practice, children and adolescents with ASD are sometimes referred for threatening to kill themselves following an argument with parents when their demands are not met. In adolescents and young adults, self-injurious behaviors such as self-cutting may be accompanied by suicidal ideation. The determination of intent to die is critical in the assessment of suicide, particularly in persons with ASD, and especially in those who are lower functioning with poor verbal skills. Despite the increase of interest in suicidal behavior in persons with ASD, few systematic studies have examined this issue in persons with intellectual disability and ASD.

Psychosis
Psychotic behavior may be defined as a disorder of thought, perception, or both. Bipolar disorder, especially in its classic form, may lead to psychotic behavior both in its depressed and in its elated phase.[12]

Catatonia
Some autistic patients who initially present with bipolar disorder gradually develop symptoms of catatonia, a life-threatening condition whose diagnosis and recognition have increased in persons with ASD over the last decade. Such patients almost always have other comorbid disorders either preceding or accompanying the symptoms of bipolar disorder, underscoring the problems inherent in studying comorbidity in this population, as discussed later.

Assessment

Diagnosis of bipolar disorder in persons with ASD depends on the developmental history, age, and the level of functioning of the person. The medical work-up should include thyroid function tests to rule out hyperthyroidism. Family psychiatric history of bipolar disorder also increases the risk. The differential diagnosis includes ADHD, oppositional defiant disorder, and aggressive behavior/temper tantrums in children. Rating scales and structured interviews such as the Young Mania Rating Scale[13,14] can also be used in persons with ASD, although they have not been validated specifically in this population.

Treatment

The goal of treatment of bipolar disorder in autism is 2-fold: to stabilize the mood and behavior and to prevent recurrence. Stabilization of severe hypomania, mania, or of depression is best done by medications with the help of psychotherapy aimed at the cognitive and adaptive level of the affected person. Several recent reports have described the use of mood stabilizers such as anticonvulsant agents and second-generation antipsychotic medications in this population.[15] However, it is worth noting that patients who have autism and bipolar disorder may also have concomitant disorders such as epilepsy, ADHD, severe anxiety disorder, and psychosis, all of which should also be addressed. In the most severe and refractory cases, electroconvulsive therapy (ECT) needs to be considered as an option.[16] Depending on the age and the level of functioning, adjustments should be made in the school or vocational training program.

Course and Prognosis

As with the presence of any other comorbid psychiatric disorder, the presence of bipolar disorder complicates the course of autism and vice versa. It is difficult to perform systematic studies controlling for the other comorbid disorders, such as ADHD, which are usually present either with or preceding the onset of bipolar disorder in the setting of autism. In addition, level of IQ and communication skills also need to be taken into account. In a follow-up study of patients with bipolar disorder referred to a psychiatric clinic, 30 patients with Asperger syndrome and pervasive developmental disorder, not otherwise specified (PDDNOS), diagnosed according to DSM-IV, were identified. Subjects were more socially impaired than those who had bipolar disorder without Asperger syndrome and PDDNOS. However, patients with autistic disorder were excluded from the study.[17]

PSYCHOTIC DISORDERS
Defining Psychosis

Psychosis is not an easy concept to define. Although it is the core symptom of schizophrenia, it can occur in major depression, bipolar disorder, catatonia, and other conditions such as epilepsy, dementia, delirium, substance abuse, and trauma. It typically refers to a disorder of thought and/or of perception, often accompanied by a lack of insight. According to the DSM-5, which takes a narrow approach to its definition, psychosis is characterized by the presence of hallucinations without insight into their pathologic nature, delusions, or both hallucinations without insight and delusions.[18] Although thought disorder per se is not required for the diagnosis of psychosis, it can be considered a diagnostic feature in the presence of extremely disorganized behavior or severe negative symptoms.

Schizophrenia

Background
Before reviewing recent publications on the comorbidity of autism and schizophrenia, it is important to reconsider the origin of their relationship. Kanner[19] used the word autism to describe 11 children who formed the basis of his historic article. This term was derived from the work of Bleuler, who thought that autism was one of the 4 characteristic symptoms of schizophrenia, the others being ambivalence, alogia, and anhedonia.[20] Kanner[19] chose the word autism to describe the isolation and withdrawal that occurs in classic autism, and not to suggest that the 2 disorders were related. Also, the disorders were described at a time when psychoanalysis was ascendant, particularly in the practice of child psychiatry in the United States. Any severely impaired child who seemed different was called psychotic, and anyone who was psychotic was schizophrenic. Because autism, as defined in the early 1940s, was a severely handicapping condition that affected the child's development in multiple ways, it was initially labeled as infantile psychosis and later as childhood psychosis/schizophrenia. In DSM-II (1968), schizophrenia, childhood type, was classified under schizophrenia as a condition "manifested by autistic, atypical, and withdrawn behavior; failure to develop identity separate from the mother's; and general unevenness, gross immaturity and inadequacy in development."[21(p35)] It was primarily the work of Kolvin and colleagues[22] in the early 1970s in the United Kingdom that was instrumental in clarifying the differences between autism and schizophrenia,

comprehensively summarized by Michael Rutter[23] (1972). The DSM-III[24] deleted the adjective autistic in its diagnostic criteria of schizophrenia and introduced autism as the main diagnosis under pervasive developmental disorders, thus marking the separation between autism and schizophrenia. However, 40 years after the publication of DSM-III, the relationship between autism and schizophrenia continues to be controversial.

Comorbidity

One reason for the controversy is the challenge of estimating the rate of schizophrenia in persons with autism. Based on studies of narrowly defined autism, and including both high-functioning and low-functioning individuals, it is generally thought that the rate of schizophrenia in autism is the same as that in the general population. Thus, in a series of 163 patients with autism referred to a special clinic, Volkmar and Cohen[25] (1991) found only 1 patient with intellectual disability to meet the criteria for schizophrenia. Recent studies have reported much higher rates. For example, based on the Danish registry, Mouridsen and colleagues[26] reported that, in a clinic sample of 89 individuals with atypical autism, first seen as children and followed up as adults, 34.8% had at some point been diagnosed with a 'schizophrenia spectrum disorder, although atypical autism, as diagnosed by the International Statistical Classification of Diseases and Related Health Problems, Tenth Revision (ICD-10), autistic disorder, and Asperger syndrome were all included. Using the same dataset, they reported that the rate of schizophrenia in 118 subjects with infantile autism alone was 3.4%,[27] underscoring that the narrower the diagnostic criteria of autism, the lower the rate of the comorbidity between autism and schizophrenia. In a cross-sectional clinical sample of 63 high-functioning adults with ASD (DSM-IV; mean IQ, 104; mean age, 29 years), Joshi and colleagues[8] reported that the rates of lifetime and current psychosis were 8% and 5% respectively. However, psychosis is not synonymous with schizophrenia. For example, in a long-term follow-up study of 120 individuals with autism, Billstedt and colleagues[28] reported that "Eight individuals (5 males, 3 females) had been diagnosed by independent (adult) psychiatrists as suffering from psychosis. Only in one individual (male) had the psychotic condition been labelled schizophrenia." Another male patient with psychosis had a diagnosis of bipolar disorder, and "there were histories suggestive of this diagnosis in four further of those receiving a diagnosis of psychosis."[28(p356)] Thus, most of the patients in the psychosis group had a history suggestive of bipolar disorder and only 1 had been diagnosed with schizophrenia.

Similarities, Differences, and Overlap

Narrowly defined, autism is a childhood-onset disorder characterized by reciprocal social communicative deficits and restricted interests and behaviors; usually lifelong in some form; often associated with intellectual disability, other psychiatric disorders, epilepsy, and named genetic syndromes; associated with a family history of autism and related disorders; modestly responsive to behavioral and psychopharmacologic interventions; and generally marked by a less-than-optimum outcome. In contrast, schizophrenia, narrowly defined, is a late-adolescent/early adulthood–onset disorder defined by the presence of deficits of perception and thought, with no specific relationship with intellectual disability or epilepsy, although it may be overrepresented in some genetic syndromes, associated with a family history of schizophrenia and related disorders, partly responsive to pharmacologic agents, and marked by a varied outcome.[23]

Although the developmental history is critical in separating the 2 conditions, some studies have suggested that autisticlike symptoms may occur in the premorbid histories of adults with schizophrenia.[29] Although necessarily retrospective, these studies have highlighted the overlap that may occur between the 2 disorders, suggesting that they may start looking similar then follow separate trajectories or merge later resulting in a comorbidity. Some subtypes of individuals with ASDs may have first-degree relatives with schizophrenia-related disorders. A family genetic study of subjects with narrowly defined Asperger syndrome found that, of the 58 subjects, 9 (15%) had a family history of schizophrenia.[30]

Molecular genetic studies have revealed shared copy number variants, deletions, and duplications such as 22q11.2, 1q21.1, and 15q13.3, and overlapping genes such as BDNF, CHRNA7, DISC1, DRD2, suggesting that the 2 disorders may be related.[31] In addition, overlapping genes FOXP2, HTR2A, MAOA, MTHFR, SLC6A3, and TPH2 have been found to be involved both in schizophrenia and ASD. However, similar findings have been reported in other conditions, such as bipolar disorder, ADHD, and obsessive-compulsive disorder, and are not specific to the relationship between autism and schizophrenia.[10]

Although both patients with autism and with schizophrenia may have deficits of social cognition, subtle differences may exist between the 2 groups. Tobe and colleagues[32] (2016) administered a social cognition battery using both auditory and visual emotion recognition measures to a group of 19 high-functioning individuals with ASD, 92 individuals with schizophrenia, and 73 healthy control adults. Patients with schizophrenia were impaired on both auditory and visual measures, whereas patients with ASD had intact auditory function but were impaired on visual emotion measure only.

Mentalizing deficits, which index the impairment of the ability to infer the mental states of others, have been reported in both disorders. Based on a meta-analysis of 37 studies, Chung and colleagues[33] investigated whether differences in clinical features of the 2 disorders predicted different patterns of performance on mentalizing tests. They concluded that adults with schizophrenia showed a trend toward greater impairments on verbal than on visual mentalizing tasks, whereas adults with ASD did not show different levels of impairment on the verbal versus visual tasks. In an imaging study, Toal and colleagues[34] (2009) compared 14 adults with ASD with psychosis, 16 without psychosis, and 16 healthy controls. The ASD groups had increased gray matter in the striatal region but less in both the temporal lobes and the cerebellum, but those with comorbid psychosis also had reduced gray matter in the frontal and occipital regions, right insular cortex, and bilaterally in the cerebellum, and reduced white matter in the cerebellum and the left lingual gyrus. Because these abnormalities differed from those reported in psychosis in general and resembled those tentatively reported in at-risk studies of psychosis in young persons, the investigators suggested that the results might represent an alternative entry point into a final common pathway of psychosis.

Assessment

Diagnosing schizophrenia in autism depends on the age of the patient, the subtype of the disorder, the presence of intellectual disability, the level of verbal skills, and the presence of other comorbid disorders. Because there is no biological test for the diagnosis of either autism or schizophrenia, the diagnosis remains clinical; rating scales and structured interviews only provide supplementary information. If an autistic child has severe intellectual disability with impaired speech, it is virtually impossible to make a confident diagnosis of schizophrenia. Between the ages of 5 and 12 years, children with autism with good verbal skills sometimes report seeing and hearing things that do not exist. However, these reports must be carefully distinguished from illusions, overvalued ideas, misinterpretations, imaginary ideas, autistic fixations and persever-ations, delayed echolalia, and so forth. If an adolescent aged between 13 and 18 years complains of symptoms suggestive of auditory and visual hallucinations, the differen-tial diagnosis should then include depression and substance abuse disorders, which are much more common than schizophrenia in the general population. If an adult with autism and severe intellectual disability is suspected of psychosis, then the assess-ment should be based on techniques used in persons with intellectual disability. How-ever, in high-functioning individuals with autism, the assessment should be based on tools used in the general population. In contrast, ruling out autism in an adult with an established diagnosis of schizophrenia or psychosis presents its own challenges. The diagnosis depends on eliciting a credible developmental history, which is not always possible. The distinction is particularly difficult in patients who have negative symp-toms of schizophrenia because of the resemblance with the aloof and passive social subtypes of ASDs.

Treatment

The main objective is to stabilize the patient and ensure the safety of others. There are no specific medications that target the core symptoms of autism in general or in the presence of psychosis. Treatment of autism and psychotic behavior is essentially symptomatic. If the psychosis is secondary to another disorder, such as a severe mood disorder or substance abuse, or catatonia, that disorder should also be treated. Antipsychotic medications such as Risperdal are commonly used in patients with and without autism. Other drugs used in the treatment of schizophrenia have also been used in autism in open studies, such as Clozaril, oxytocin, and bumetanide.[35,36] In re-fractory cases, ECT may be considered.[37] In addition, supportive and cognitive behavior psychotherapy, along with providing support to the family, should be pro-vided depending on the clinical status of the patient. Although outcome studies of autism have not systematically studied the role of psychosis, there is clinical evidence that comorbidity in general negatively affects the long-term prognosis.

DISCLOSURE

The authors have nothing to disclose.

REFERENCES

1. American Psychiatric Association. Diagnostic and statistical manual of mental disorders-5th edition (DSM-5) 2013. Washington, DC.
2. Ghaziuddin M. Mental health aspects of autism and asperger syndrome. Phila-delphia: Jessica Kingsley Press; 2005. p. 134–5.
3. Wozniak J, Biederman J, Faraone S, et al. Mania in children with pervasive devel-opmental disorder revisited. J Am Acad Child Adolesc Psychiatry 1997;36(11):1552–9.
4. Vannucchi G, Masi G, Toni C, et al. Bipolar disorder in adults with Asperger' s syndrome: a systematic review. J Affect Disord 2014;168:151–60.
5. Munesue T, Ono Y, Mutoh K, et al. High prevalence of bipolar disorder comorbid-ity in adolescents and young adults with high-functioning autism spectrum disor-der: a preliminary study of 44 outpatients. J Affect Disord 2008;111(2–3):170–5.
6. Gutkovich Z, Carlson G, Carlson H, et al. Asperger's disorder and co-morbid bi-polar disorder: diagnostic and treatment challenges. J Child Adolesc Psycho-pharmacol 2007;7(2):247–56.

7. Sapmaz D, Baykal S, Akbaş S. The clinical features of comorbid pediatric bipolar disorder in children with autism spectrum disorder. J Autism Dev Disord 2018; 48(8):2800–8.

8. Joshi G, Biederman J, Petty C, et al. Examining the comorbidity of bipolar disorder and autism spectrum disorders: a large controlled analysis of phenotypic and familial correlates in a referred population of youth with bipolar i disorder with and without autism spectrum disorders. J Clin Psychiatry 2013;74(6):578–86.

9. Morgan V, Croft M, Valuri G, et al. Intellectual disability and other neuropsychiatric outcomes in high-risk children of mothers with schizophrenia, bipolar disorder and unipolar major depression. Br J Psychiatry 2012;200(4):282–9.

10. O'Connell K, McGregor N, Lochner C, et al. The genetic architecture of schizophrenia, bipolar disorder, obsessive-compulsive disorder and autism spectrum disorder. Mol Cell Neurosci 2018;88:300–7.

11. Weissman A, Bates M. Increased clinical and neurocognitive impairment in children with autism spectrum disorders and comorbid bipolar disorder. Res Autism Spectr Disord 2010;4(4):670–80.

12. Selten J, Lundberg M, Rai D, et al. Risks for nonaffective psychotic disorder and bipolar disorder in young people with autism spectrum disorder: a population-based study. JAMA Psychiatry 2015;72(5):483–9.

13. Young R, Biggs J, Ziegler V, et al. A rating scale for mania: reliability, validity and sensitivity. Br J Psychiatry 1978;(133):429–35.

14. Youngstrom E, Gracious B, Danielson C, et al. Toward an integration of parent and clinician report on the Young Mania Rating Scale. J Affect Disord 2003; 77(2):179–90.

15. Joshi G, Biederman J, Wozniak J, et al. Response to second generation antipsychotics in youth with comorbid bipolar disorder and autism spectrum disorder. CNS Neurosci Ther 2012;18(1):28–33.

16. Siegel M, Milligan B, Robbins D, et al. Electroconvulsive therapy in an adolescent with autism and bipolar I disorder. J ECT 2012;28(4):252–5.

17. Borue X, Mazefsky C, Rooks B, et al. Longitudinal course of bipolar disorder in youth with high-functioning autism spectrum disorder. J Am Acad Child Adolesc Psychiatry 2016;55(12):1064–72.

18. American Psychiatric Association. DSM-5 task force. Diagnostic and statistical manual of mental disorders: DSM-5. 5th edition. Washington, DC: American Psychiatric Association; 2013.

19. Kanner L. Autistic disturbances of affective contact. Nervous Child 1943;2(3): 100–36.

20. Fusar-Poli P, Politi P. Paul Eugen Bleuler and the birth of schizophrenia (1908). Am J Psychiatry 2008;165(11):1407.

21. American Psychiatric Association. Committee on nomenclature and statistics. Diagnostic and statistical manual of mental disorders, DSM II (second edition). 2nd edition. Washington, DC: American Psychiatric Association; 1968.

22. Kolvin I, Ounsted C, Humphrey M, et al. The phenomenology of childhood psychoses. Br J Psychiatry 1971;118:385–95.

23. Rutter M. Childhood schizophrenia reconsidered. J Autism Child Schizophr 1972; 2(4):313–37.

24. Volkmar F, Cicchetti D, Bregman J, et al. Three diagnostic systems for autism: DSM-III, DSM-III-R, ICD-10. J Autism Dev Disord 1992;22(4):483–92.

25. Volkmar F, Cohen D. Comorbid association of autism and schizophrenia. Am J Psychiatry 1991;148(12):1705–7.

26. Mouridsen SE, Rich B, Isager T. Psychiatric disorders in adults diagnosed as children with atypical autism. A case control study. J Neural Transm 2008;115(1): 135–8.
27. Mouridsen S, Rich B, Isager T, et al. Psychiatric disorders in individuals diagnosed with infantile autism as children: a case control study. J Psychiatr Pract 2008;14(1):5–12.
28. Billstedt E, Gillberg C, Gillberg C. Autism after adolescence: population-based 13-to 22-year follow-up study of 120 individuals with autism diagnosed in childhood. J Autism Dev Disord 2005;35(3):351–60.
29. McKenna K, Gordon C, Lenane M, et al. Looking for childhood-onset schizophrenia: the first 71 cases screened. J Am Acad Child Adolesc Psychiatry 1994;33(5):177–82.
30. Ghaziuddin M. A family history study of Asperger syndrome. J Autism Dev Disord 2005;35(2):177–82.
31. Zheng Z, Zheng P, Zou X. Association between schizophrenia and autism spectrum disorder: a systematic review and meta analysis. Autism Res 2018;11(8): 1110–9.
32. Tobe R, Corcoran C, Breland M, et al. Differential profiles in auditory social cognition deficits between adults with autism and schizophrenia spectrum disorders: a preliminary analysis. J Psychiatr Res 2016;1(79):21–7.
33. Chung Y, Barch D, Strube M. A meta-analysis of mentalizing impairments in adults with schizophrenia and autism spectrum disorder. Schizophr Bull 2013; 40(3):602–16.
34. Toal F, Bloemen O, Deeley Q, et al. Psychosis and autism: magnetic resonance imaging study of brain anatomy. Br J Psychiatry 2009;194(5):418–25.
35. LeClerc S, Easley D. Pharmacological therapies for autism spectrum disorder: a review. P T 2015;40(6):418–25.
36. Ji N, Findling R. An update on pharmacotherapy for autism spectrum disorder in children and adolescents. Curr Opin Psychiatry 2015;28(2):91–101.
37. Ghaziuddin N, Kutcher SP, Knapp P, American Academy of Child and Adolescent Psychiatry Work Group on Quality Issues. Summary of the practice parameter for the use of electroconvulsive therapy with adolescents. J Am Acad Child Adolesc Psychiatry 2004;43(1):119–22.

Catatonia in Patients with Autism Spectrum Disorder

Neera Ghaziuddin, MD, MRCPsych(UK)[a,*], Laura Andersen, MD[b],
Mohammad Ghaziuddin, MD[a]

KEYWORDS

- Catatonia • Autism • Asperger syndrome

KEY POINTS

- Catatonia is a severe psychiatric disorder that can occur in persons with autism spectrum disorders (ASD).
- Common symptoms include changes in motor function, reduced or loss of speech, decline in previously acquired skill level, and other psychiatric symptoms.
- Symptoms of catatonia usually appear during adolescence and early adulthood, but may emerge at different times across the life span of a person with autism.
- Persons with ASD are probably at an increased risk of developing this condition compared with the general population.
- The only known current treatments are benzodiazepines and/or electroconvulsive therapy. The diagnosis, treatment, and outcome are complicated by the co-occurrence of other medical and psychiatric symptoms.

 Video content accompanies this article at http://www.childpsych.theclinics. com.

INTRODUCTION

Catatonia is a relatively common and a serious neuropsychiatric syndrome that can occur in patients with autism spectrum disorder (ASD) and in a variety of other psychiatric and medical disorders. The history of catatonia is important because a revised understanding has resulted in considerable changes in its treatment. The condition was first described by Karl Ludwig Kahlbaum in 1874, who defined it as a motor syndrome occurring in association with affective disorders, epilepsy, and tuberculosis.[1] In

This article originally appeared in *Child and Adolescent Psychiatric Clinics*, Volume 29, Issue 3, July 2020.

[a] University of Michigan, University of Michigan Medical Center, 4250 Plymouth Road, Ann Arbor, MI 48109, USA; [b] Department of Psychiatry, University of Michigan, 1500 E Medical Center Drive, Ann Arbor, MI 48108, USA
* Corresponding author.
E-mail address: neerag@umich.edu

psych.theclinics.com

its initial description, Kahlbaum had specifically noted that the condition should not be confused with "degeneration,"[2] which was later renamed as schizophrenia by Bleuler in 1911. However, 2 prominent nineteenth century psychiatrists of the time, Kraepelin and Bleuler, classified catatonia with schizophrenia.[3,4] This misclassification persisted over the subsequent100 years, and was explained using psychodynamic theories,[5] psychosocial concepts such as institutionalization,[6] and as side effects of antipsychotic agents.[7] It was only with the publication of the *Diagnostic and Statistical Manual of Mental Disorders, 5th Edition: DSM-5* (DSM-5) in 2013, and after much lobbying by experts,[8] that catatonia was finally recognized in a variety of psychiatric and medical disorders instead of being considered as a subtype of schizophrenia. Many experts have suggested that catatonia should be recognized as a stand-alone syndrome, or sui generis (unique).

There are historical reports of catatonia noted in children and adolescents with autism.[9,10] However, starting in the 1990s, catatonia comorbid with autism and its treatment with benzodiazepines and electroconvulsive therapy (ECT) were finally recognized.[11–14] Although controversial, some have even proposed that in selected cases, autism may be an early expression of catatonia.[15,16]

CATATONIA IN THE DIAGNOSTIC AND STATISTICAL MANUAL OF MENTAL DISORDERS

The most notable change in the nosology of catatonia resulted with the publication of DSM-5 in 2013. These changes have been summarized by Tandon and colleagues,[17] and include the following: first, catatonia is no longer recognized as a subtype of schizophrenia; second, uniform criteria across diagnoses are advised for identifying catatonia, which unlike DSM-IV, allowed using different criteria depending on whether a patient was diagnosed with a co-occurring mood disorder, schizophrenia, or a medical condition; third, 3 symptoms are now necessary to make the diagnosis, versus only 2 symptoms required in DSM-IV; and last, a new category of catatonia not otherwise specified (catatonia-NOS) has been added, which allows this diagnosis to be made when an underlying cause is not known.[17]

PREVALENCE

Catatonia has been reported in a range of psychiatric disorders; however, it is not known whether individuals with ASD may have a greater susceptibility. Relatively high rates of catatonia have been reported in both ASD and in non-ASD patient groups. For instance, 16.9% were identified among hospitalized patients with psychosis,[18] 13.5% were identified in India, and 9.6% in Wales among consecutively admitted patients to acute psychiatry units,[19] and 24% were found among patients with comorbid delirium.[20]

In one of the earliest systematic examinations, among 506 patients with ASD compared with controls, Wing and Shah[13] found that17% had symptoms of catatonia among patients 15 years or older, approximately. Most of their patients were male (male patients = 28, female patients = 2), the onset of catatonia was most common in age range 10 to 19 years, no precipitants could be identified in most, and there was no statistical difference in the rates of seizure disorders between the ASD group with catatonia versus those without catatonia (13% vs 22%).[13] In a subsequent study, the investigators also reported learning disability and intellectual disability as additional risk factors for developing catatonia.[21] Ghaziuddin and colleagues[22] studied hospitalized patients with a range of diagnoses (ASD, psychosis NOS, intermittent explosive disorder) and found that 17.8% of the participants met criteria for catatonia;

however, only a single patient among the 18 identified had been accurately labeled. Study findings underscored a male preponderance, underdiagnosis of catatonia even in highly specialized psychiatric settings, high rates of aggression, and an association with intellectual disability.[22]

Catatonia with ASD has been associated with chromosomal and genetic disorders. These include Phelan McDermid syndrome,[23] Prader-Willi syndrome,[24] and 22q11.2 deletion syndrome.[25] Catatonia also has been described in Down syndrome, which may be associated with autism in some cases, although the frequency is unknown.[26–28] Therefore, a high index of suspicion is recommended when treating patients with ASD with these coexisting genetic disorders.

ETIOLOGY

The pathophysiology underlying catatonia remains unclear, although there are several proposed factors, including neurotransmitter-related, infective, genetic, immunologic, metabolic, and psychological. Gamma-aminobutyric acid (GABA) has been proposed as a common pathway, and other hypotheses include seizures, which are associated with both conditions, reduced density of GABA receptors, and a genetic vulnerability as defined by diagnosable syndromes.

The GABA hypothesis is primarily supported by a positive response to GABA receptor modulators, such as benzodiazepines[15,29–31]; patients being able to tolerate relatively high dosages of benzodiazepines without experiencing sedation; and a positive response to other GABA agonists, such as zolpidem and ECT.[30,31] Seizure disorders are suggested as another common pathway, which are found in both autism and catatonia, with up to a third of patients with autism having a seizure disorder.[32] However, patients with ASD and catatonia, compared with those without catatonia, have similar rates of a seizure disorder.[13] Neuroimaging has provided evidence of decreased $GABA_A$ receptor density found in the left sensorimotor cortex in akinetic catatonia.[33,34] Regarding clinical comorbidity, catatonia in ASD appears to be associated with psychosis,[35] where ECT can be particularly helpful[36] with mood disorders[14] and in some patients with tic disorders and obsessive-compulsive disorder (OCD).[37,38]

A number of infective and inflammatory conditions may be associated with catatonia, suggesting an immunologic etiology for catatonia. Examples include bacterial or viral meningitis or encephalitis, other systemic infections, and autoimmune disorders, including autoimmune thyroid disorders, encephalitis, and demyelinating disorders.[39] N-methyl-D-aspartate (NMDA) encephalitis associated with catatonia has been reported in patients with autism and intellectual disability, raising the question of whether there is an underlying vulnerability in this population.[40]

Finally, trauma, severe stress, and grief may precipitate catatonia, which was originally described by Kahlbaum.[41] It has been suggested that individuals with autism may be particularly vulnerable to stress, given their cognitive and social limitations.[42]

SIGNS AND SYMPTOMS

Key symptoms of catatonia can be identified under 3 clinical domains, namely *motor, speech,* and *behavioral.* Symptoms should be either a new-onset or a considerable worsening of preexisting symptoms.[13,14] Onset appears to be acute with a waxing and waning course[43] and often coincides with the onset of puberty with a relatively high rate seen between 10 and 19 years.[13] DSM-5 diagnostic criteria require 3 of 12 symptoms, irrespective of the presence of another psychiatric disorder or a medical condition, or if the catatonia is of unspecified etiology. Symptoms included in DSM-5 are stupor, catalepsy, waxy flexibility, mutism, negativism, posturing, mannerism, stereotypy, agitation, grimacing, echolalia, and echopraxia.[44] However, according to some experts, up to 40 different symptoms of catatonia have been described in the literature,[43] which underscores the risk of overlooking the diagnosis when strictly applying the DSM-5 criteria.

Motor signs may include a change in the overall activity level (extreme hypoactivity, hyperactivity, or a mixed picture with alternating increased and reduced activity), unusual movements (posturing, mannerisms, stereotypies - a movement that is abnormal due to its frequency, grimacing, reduced eye-blink rate resulting in a staring gaze, and tics), changes in muscle tone (catalepsy or a sudden loss of muscle tone, a candle-wax–like muscle tone known as waxiflexibility, increased or reduced muscle tone), changes in handwriting, and gait changes. In severe cases, the patient may develop stupor. Based on the overall change in the motor activity level, excited or psychomotor retardation, catatonia has been broadly divided into an excited and a retarded subtype.[45] Self-injurious behavior, which is completely or partially unresponsive to environmental cues is also considered a motor stereotypy and a symptom of catatonia in people with autism or other developmental disabilities.[46] High rates of catatonia symptoms (87%) have been identified in Tourette syndrome.[47] Chorea has been noted in a small number of patients diagnosed with catatonia.[48] Speech changes may include mutism in extreme cases, reduced overall speech, verbigeration (incomprehensible speech), perseveration (repetition of a phrase or a word), or verbal stereotypies (senseless repetition of sounds or words).[44,49]

Behavioral symptoms are invariably present and may include regression or a decline in skill level (social, academic, activities of daily living), mood symptoms, repetitive behaviors resembling OCD, and/or bizarre behaviors (patient may spend hours in the bathroom repeatedly washing hands)[14] and thoughts resembling psychosis. In some cases, behavior symptoms such as withdrawal or depression may appear or even precede the motor and speech disturbance.[14] These behavior symptoms are rarely responsive to antidepressants, antipsychotics, or to mood stabilizers and in some cases these agents may precipitate a more fulminating clinical picture described as malignant catatonia.[50] Catatonia is rarely associated with schizophrenia, or responsive to antipsychotic treatments,[51] although psychotic symptoms associated with catatonia in autism have been frequently reported.[35]

Unusual symptoms have been anecdotally reported, such as an extreme sensitivity to range of sensory experiences (touch, taste, light, movement), which should alert clinicians for catatonia and warrant further examination. There are also reports of Capgras syndrome in catatonia with ASD. The condition is defined as a delusional belief that family members and friends have been replaced by an exact double and has been reported in a variety of neuropsychiatric conditions.[52]

Videos 1–5 and **Fig. 1** are included to demonstrate signs and symptoms of catatonia and the risk of injury to caregivers. In each case, the patient had received extensive multidisciplinary laboratory and other workup to rule out a treatable medical etiology.

ASSESSMENT AND TREATMENT
Assessment

Early assessment for catatonia is imperative for any patient with ASD who displays a notable change in behavior or functional status. At a minimum, the evaluation should include a comprehensive history, completing a standardized rating scale for catatonia, medical workup, physical examination, and a lorazepam challenge test[29,42] followed by a trial of lorazepam. Catatonia can persist for years, becoming chronic and resulting in diagnostic confusion.[53]

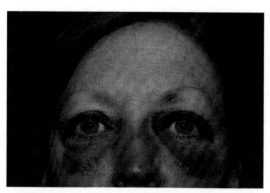

Fig. 1. Severe injury in a parent caring for a patient with ASD and catatonia. She had sustained extensive bruising and a broken nose due to unprovoked head-butting before child's treatment.

When catatonia is suspected, the initial physical examination and workup should document symptoms and exclude medical causes using basic laboratory tests, such as a complete blood count, comprehensive metabolic panel, urinalysis and culture, urine toxicology, and thyroid functions. A creatinine phosphokinase enzyme level should also be measured, followed by serial measurements, whenever there is concern for malignant catatonia or neuroleptic malignant syndrome.[50,54] Additional workup may include brain imaging, serology for autoimmune antibodies including lupus, and anti-NMDA receptors, which should be decided on a case-by-case basis and in consultation with other specialists. Electroencephalogram should be completed to rule out a seizure disorder. Standard of care is to simultaneously treat any existing medical etiology, if present, along with anti-catatonia treatments.

Catatonia rating scales are important for quantifying symptoms, measuring the symptom-severity, and to measure the treatment response longitudinally. The Bush-Francis Catatonia Scale[55] is perhaps the best known and the most widely used instrument, although several other catatonia rating scales are available, including the Northoff Catatonia Scale and the Baunig Catatonia Rating Scale.[56] These instruments have good interrater and test-retest reliability,[56] although none have been validated in patients with autism. The only exception is the Attenuated Behavior Questionnaire, which is completed by a caregiver of adolescents and young adults with an existing ASD diagnosis.[57]

The next step should include determining the severity of the illness, as described by Dhossche and colleagues[58] in the chapter "Blue prints for the assessment, treatment, and future study of catatonia in autism spectrum disorders" (**Fig. 2**). ECT is reserved for severe forms of the illness.[29,58]

Treatment

Benzodiazepines and ECT are the only known effective treatments of catatonia.[59] The speed of progressing from an unsuccessful trial of a benzodiazepine to ECT would depend on the severity of the illness. The most commonly used benzodiazepine is lorazepam, which may be administered initially as a test dose in a patient who does not have life-threatening symptoms (unable to eat or drink, unstable vital signs, concern for organ failure, uncontrollable agitation). Generally, catatonia improves considerably after a 1-mg or 2gmg test dose of lorazepam, taken orally or via intramuscular route. Lorazepam should be titrated up as best tolerated and continued for an extended

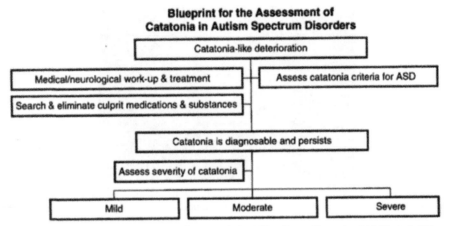

Fig. 2. Blueprint for the assessment of catatonia in ASDs. (*From* Dhossche DM, Shah A, Wing L. Blueprints for the assessment, treatment, and future study of catatonia in autism spectrum disorders. Int Rev Neurobiol 2006;72:270; with permission.)

period (months or even years) in patients who respond. Daily dosages may range from 10 to 24 mg[29]; however, higher dosages have been reported. Surprisingly, high dosages in catatonic patients, unlike in patients without catatonia, are not associated with sedating side effects, possibly reflecting a dysfunction of the GABA or the GABA-benzodiazepine receptors.[30,31] An alternative to lorazepam is zolpidem, 5 to 10 mg, which is available only in oral form.[42] It is important to note that a negative response to lorazepam does not rule out catatonia and both lack of response and deterioration have been reported in patients with ASD. For instance, Wachtel[60] reported that among 22 cases diagnosed with ASD and catatonia, most did not have a positive response to lorazepam. A failed lorazepam or an amobarbital challenge test also has been reported among 20% of general psychiatric patients and should not be regarded as a reason to rule out a catatonia diagnosis.[61,62] Therefore, based on the current knowledge, it appears that patients with catatonia and ASD may experience a markedly less robust response to lorazepam, and possibly to a lorazepam challenge test.

Bilateral ECT is the preferred mode,[59] and should be considered in patients who either do not respond to a benzodiazepine or display serious and/or life-threatening symptoms (refusal or inability to eat or drink, intense agitation, aggression including self-injurious behavior, neuroleptic malignant syndrome/malignant catatonia). The index ECT course often needs to be prolonged (a standard index course of 12 treatments is rarely effective), and similarly prolonged maintenance ECT, over months or even years, is often necessary to avoid relapse.[29,60,63] The American Academy of Child and Adolescent Psychiatry guidelines recommend a consensus of 3 child psychiatrists when ECT is considered for a minor patient, although this requirement may vary by state in the United States.[64] In some instances, this requirement for consensus may prevent timely access to ECT because many child and adolescent psychiatrists are unfamiliar with its use.[65-67] Concerns about the effect of maintenance ECT on neurodevelopment and memory are relatively common, but objective testing and follow-up studies have demonstrated stability in academic performance and cognitive functions.[68] However, there is a paucity of studies of patients with ASD treated with ECT, due to comorbid cognitive limitations. The reader is referred to the article on ECT by Sa Eun Park's article, "Use of Electroconvulsive Therapy in

Autism," elsewhere in this issue, for further details. **Fig. 3** provides the essentials of a treatment algorithm.

There is no evidence to support the use of antipsychotic or antidepressant medications in patients with catatonia who present with psychotic or affective symptoms. Both the emergence of catatonia in patients receiving antipsychotic agents,[69] and a lack of response in already diagnosed patients has been reported.[22,70] Patients with catatonia also may be at risk for developing neuroleptic malignant syndrome when treated with antipsychotic agents.[22] A case-by-case determination may be made for introducing these agents after the catatonia has been successfully treated and deemed necessary.

COMPLICATIONS AND OUTCOME

Patients with ASD and catatonia are at an increased risk for negative outcomes with a 60-fold increase in mortality, which may include suicide.[71] Cornic and colleagues[71] followed 31 adolescents (ASD = 5) with catatonia over a 4-year period, whose age ranged from 12 to 18 years and found a high rate of chronicity in the entire group (8 of 31; 25%), need for ongoing psychiatric care (14 of 31; 45%), and premature death (3 of 31; 9.6%); 2 of these deaths were due to suicide. Clearly, catatonia is associated with high rates of morbidity and mortality.

Medical complications are relatively common in patients with catatonia.[72] However, because of a lack of systematic studies involving ASD, it is not known if this

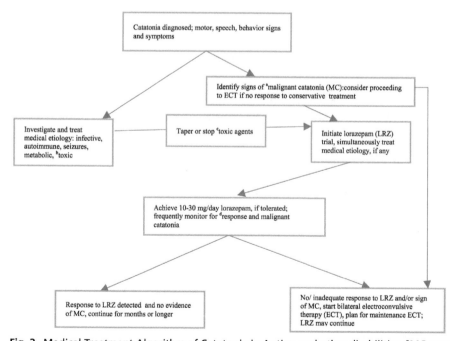

Fig. 3. Medical Treatment Algorithm of Catatonia in Autism and other disabilities. [a]MC may include abrupt change in mental status, rising creatinine phosphate enzyme, autonomic changes and fever; [b]Toxic agents may include antipsychotic (AP), antidepressants or others; [c]Unless there is MC, when rapid taper is needed, some agents such as APs may be slowly tapered; [d]Treatment response should be measured using a standardized rating scale such as Bush Francis Catatonia scale and overall clinical assessment.

patient-group may be at a higher risk for complications. Known complications may include poor nutrition, dehydration (may require enteral feeding; see case KE described later in this article), aspiration and pneumonia, poor dentition, urinary retention and infections,[73] skin breakdown and muscle contractures, and poor menstrual hygiene. The most feared complication, associated with a high mortality, is malignant catatonia, which may be precipitated by antipsychotic medications[50] or occur even when no medication can be identified. It was first described by Stauder in 1934,[74] who labeled it as fatal catatonia. The condition is almost identical to neuroleptic malignant syndrome (NMS), delirious mania, Bell mania, toxic serotonin syndrome, fulminating psychosis, and oneirophrenia.[75] Fink and Taylor[43] provide a detailed argument why NMS and malignant catatonia are identical conditions that require urgent lifesaving treatment with a benzodiazepine and/or ECT.

CASE REPORT (GASTROINTESTINAL COMPLICATIONS)

KE is a 19-year-old man with autism who resides in an intact family. Trauma, abuse, or neglect are denied. He had presented 2 years earlier when he was diagnosed with catatonia based on multiple motor symptoms (periodic immobility and agitation, posturing and freezing, impulsivity, mannerisms), speech changes (mute, echolalia), echopraxia, stereotyped behaviors (repetitive vomiting), negativism, waxiflexibility, gagenhalten, ambitendency, self-injurious behaviors, and autonomic abnormalities. His Bush-Francis Catatonia Rating score = 33. Because of declining oral intake, despite lorazepam 8 mg/d, a gastrostomy tube was placed and lorazepam was further increased, but he continued to deteriorate. Gastrointestinal workup was negative and included esophagogastroduodenoscopy, gastric emptying scan, and computed tomography abdominal scan. Neurology workup for spasms and tremors found a mild encephalopathy. Unsuccessful medication trials included fluoxetine and aripiprazole (for a presumptive OCD diagnosis), sulfamethoxazole and trimethoprim for cellulitis (likely due to reduced mobility), fluconazole for candida infection (likely due to long-term antibiotic use), cyproheptadine to improve appetite (resulted in uncontrollable mouth movements and biting of the buccal mucosa), and mixed salt amphetamine, methylphenidate, and chlorpromazine for unclear reasons. ECT with bilateral electrode placement was eventually initiated due to uncontrollable vomiting, progressive weight loss, a range of motor symptoms, and severe self-injurious behaviors. Patient is currently stable (no agitation, absent self-injurious behavior or vomiting, and variably able to accept 50%–90% of caloric intake by mouth) while receiving maintenance ECT for the past 2 years.

SUMMARY

Catatonia is a relatively common condition in ASD. It is essential that this condition is included in the differential diagnosis of patients with autism, so that it is identified and appropriately treated with a benzodiazepine alone or along with ECT. These anti-catatonic treatments have life-changing and lifesaving implications. Larger, systematic studies are necessary to better identify and treat the condition.

ACKNOWLEDGMENTS

This work was supported by Richard Tam Foundation, University of Michigan, Depression Center.

DISCLOSURE

N. Ghaziuddin: Royalties from book, *Use of Electroconvulsive Therapy in Children and Adolescents*. Publisher: Oxford University Press, 2013. M. Ghaziuddin and L. Andersen do not have any disclosures.

SUPPLEMENTARY DATA

Supplementary data related to this article can be found online at https://doi.org/10.1016/j.chc.2020.03.001.

REFERENCES

1. Barnes MP, Saunders M, Walls TJ, et al. The syndrome of Karl Ludwig Kahlbaum. J Neurol Neurosurg Psychiatry 1986;49(9).
2. Gelenberg A. The Catatonia syndrome. Lancet 1976;1(7973):1339–41.
3. Kraepelin E. Dementia praecox and paraphrenia. Edinburgh (United Kingdom): E & S Livingstone; 1919.
4. Blueler E. Dementia praecox or the group of schizophrenias (Zinkin J, trans). New York: International Universities Press; 1950.
5. Rogers D. Catatonia: a contemporary approach. J Neuropsychiatry 1991;3(3): 334–40.
6. Johnson J. Catatonia: the tension insanity. Br J Psychiatry 1993;162:733–8.
7. Clark T, Rickards H. Catatonia 1: history and clinical features. Hosp Med 1990; 60(10):740–2.
8. Francis A, Fink M, Appiani F, et al. Catatonia in DSM5. J ECT 2010;26(4):246–7.
9. Maudsley H. Insanity of early life.. In: Maudsley H, editor. The phsysiology and pathology of the mind. New York: Appleton; 1867. p. 442.
10. Creek M. Schizophrenic syndrome in childhood: further progress report of a working party. Dev Med Child Neurol 1964;4:530–5.
11. Realmuto GM, August GJ. Catatonia in autistic disorder: a sign of comorbidity or variable expression? J Autism Dev Disord 1991;21(4):517–28.
12. Dhossche D. Brief report: catatonia in autistic disorder. J Autism Dev Disord 1998;28(4):329–31.
13. Wing L, Shah A. Catatonia in autistic spectrum disorders. Br J Psychiatry 2000; 176:357–62 [see comment].
14. Ghaziuddin M, Quinlan P, Ghaziuddin N. Catatonia in autism: a distinct subtype? J Intellect Disabil Res 2005;49(Pt 1):102–5.
15. Dhossche DM. Autism as early expression of catatonia. Med Sci Monit 2004; 10(3):RA31–9.
16. Hare D, Malone C. Catatonia and autistic spectrum disorders. Autism 2004;8(2): 183–95.
17. Tandon R, Heckers S, Bustillo J, et al. Catatonia in DSM 5. Schizophr Res 2013; 150(1):26–30.
18. Peralta V, Cuesta M, Serrana J, et al. The Kahlbaum syndrome: a study of its clinical validity, nosological status and relationship with schizophrenia and mood disorder. Compr Psychiatry 1997;38(1):61–7.
19. Chalasani PH, Healy D, Morris R. Presentation and frequency of catatonia in new admissions to acute psychiatric admission units in India and Wales. Psychol Med 2005;35(11):1667–75.

20. Wilson JE, Carlson R, Duggan MC, et al. Delirium and catatonia in critically ill patients: the DeCat prospective cohort investigation. Crit Care Med 2017;45(11): 1837–44.
21. Wing L, Shah A. A systematic examination of catatonia-like clinical pictures in autism spectrum disorders. Int Rev Neurobiol 2006;72:21.
22. Ghaziuddin N, Dhossche D, Marcotte K. Retrospective chart review of catatonia in child and adolescent psychiatric patients. Acta Psychiatr Scand 2012; 125:33–8.
23. Serret S, Thummler S, Dor E, et al. Lithium as a rescue therapy for regression and catatonia features in two SHANK3 patients with autism spectrum disorder: case reports. BMC Psychiatry 2015;15:107.
24. Dhossche DM, Song Y, Liu Y. Is there a connection between autism, Prader-Willi syndrome, catatonia, and GABA? Int Rev Neurobiol 2005;71:189–216.
25. Butcher N, Boot E, Lang A, et al. Neuropsychiatric expression and catatonia in 22q.2 deletion syndrome: an overview and case series. Am J Med Genet 2018; 176(10):2146–56.
26. Ghaziuddin M, Tsai L, Ghaziuddin N. Autism in Down's syndrome: presentation and diagnosis. J Intellect Disabil Res 1992;36:449–56.
27. Miles J, Takahashi N, Muckerman J, et al. Catatonia in Down syndrome: systematic approach to diagnosis, treatment and outcome assessment based on a case series of seven patients. Neuropsychiatr Dis Treat 2019;15:2723–41.
28. Ghaziuddin N, Nassiri A, Miles J. Catatonia in Down syndrome. Neuropsychiatr Dis Treat 2015;11:941–9.
29. Fink M, Taylor MA, Ghaziuddin N. Catatonia in autistic spectrum disorders: a medical treatment algorithm. Int Rev Neurobiol 2006;72:233–44.
30. Dhossche D, Stoppelbein L, Rout U. Etiopathogenesis of catatonia; generalizations and working hypotheses. J ECT 2010;26(4):253–8.
31. Daniels J. Catatonia: clinical aspects and neurolbiological correlates. J Neuropsychiatry Clin Neurosci 2009;21(4):371–80.
32. Fink M, Taylor MA. Catatonia: subtype or syndrome in DSM? [see comment]. Am J Psychiatry 2006;163(11):1875–6.
33. Northoff G, Steinke R, Czcervenka C, et al. Decreased density of GABA-A receptors in the left sensorimotor cortex in akinetic catatonia: investigation of in vivo benzodiazepine receptor binding. J Neurol Neurosurg Psychiatry 1999;67(4): 445–50.
34. Walther S, Stegmayer K, Wilson J, et al. Structure and neural mechanisms of catatonia. Lancet Psychiatry 2019;6:610–9.
35. Shorter E, Wachtel L. Childhood catatonia, autism and psychosis past and present: is there an "iron triangle"? Acta Psychiatr Scand 2013;128(1):21–33.
36. Wachtel L, Schuldt S, Ghaziuddin N, et al. The potential role of electroconvulsive therapy in the "Iron Triangle" of pediatric catatonia, autism, and psychosis. Acta Psychiatr Scand 2013;128(5):408–9.
37. Bejerot S. An autistic dimension: a proposed subtype of obsessive-compulsive disorder. Autism 2007;11(2):101–10.
38. Dhosche D, Reti I, Shettar S, et al. Tics as signs of catatonia: electroconvulsive therapy response in 2 men. J ECT 2010;26(4):266–9.
39. Rogers J, Pollak T, Blackman G, et al. Catatonia and the immune system: a review. Lancet Psychiatry 2019;6:620–30.
40. Kiani R, Lawden M, Eames P, et al. Anti-NMDA-receptor encephalitis presenting with catatonia and neuroleptic malignant syndrome in patients with intellectual disability and autism. BJPsych Bull 2015;39:32–5.

41. Dhossche D, Ross C, Stoppelbein L. The role of deprivation, abuse, trauma in pediatric catatonia without a clear medical cause. Acta Psychiatr Scand 2012; 125(1):25–32.

42. Dhossche D, Withane N. Electroconvulsive therapy for catatonia in children and adolescents. Child Adolesc Psychiatr Clin N Am 2019;28:111–20.

43. Fink M, Taylor MA. The many varieties of catatonia. Eur Arch Psychiatry Clin Neurosci 2001;251(Suppl 1):I8–13.

44. American Psychiatric Association. American Psychiatric Association. DSM-5 Task Force. *Diagnostic and statistical manual of mental disorders: DSM-5*. 5th edition. Washington, DC: American Psychiatric Association; 2013.

45. Morrison J. Catatonia: retarded and excited types. Arch Gen Psychiatry 1973; 28(1):39–41.

46. Wachtel LE, Dhossche DM. Self-injury in autism as an alternate sign of catatonia: implications for electroconvulsive therapy. Med Hypotheses 2010;75(1):111–4.

47. Cavanna A. Catatonic signs in Gilles de la Tourette syndrome. Cogn Behav Neurol 2008;21(1):34–7.

48. Consoli A, Raffin M, Laurent C, et al. Medical and developmental risk factors for catatonia in children and adolescents: a prospective case-control study. Schizophr Res 2012;137(1–3):151–8.

49. Ghaziuddin M. Mental health aspects of autism and Asperger syndrome. Philadelphia: Jessica Kingsley Publishers; 2005.

50. Ghaziuddin N, Hendriks M, Patel P, et al. Neuroleptic malignant syndrome/Malignant catatonia in child psychiatry: literature review and a case series. J Child Adolesc Psychiatry 2017;27(4):359–65.

51. Abrams R, Taylor MA. Catatonia. A prospective clinical study. Arch Gen Psychiatry 1976;33(5):579–81.

52. Josephs K. Capgras syndrome and its relationship to neurodegenerative disease. Arch Neurol 2007;64:1762–6.

53. Ghaziuddin N, Gih D, Barbosa V, et al. Onset of catatonia at puberty: electroconvulsive therapy response in two autistic adolescents. J ECT 2010;26(4):274–7.

54. Ghaziuddin N, Alkhouri I, Champine D, et al. ECT treatment of malignant catatonia/NMS in an adolescent: a useful lesson in delayed diagnosis and treatment. J ECT 2002;18(2):95–8.

55. Bush G, Fink M, Petrides G, et al. Catatonia. I. Rating scale and standardized examination. Acta Psychiatr Scand 1996;93(2):129–36.

56. Sienaert P, Rooseleer J, De Fruyt J. Measuring catatonia: a systematic review of rating scales. J Affect Disord 2011;135(1–3):1–9.

57. Breen J, Hare D. The nature and prevalence of catatonic symptoms in young people with autism. J Intellect Disabil Res 2017;61(6):580–93.

58. Dhossche D, Shah A, Wing L. Blueprints for the assessment, treatment, and future study of catatonia in autism spectrum disorders. In: Dhossche D, Wing L, Ohta M, et al, editors. Catatonia in autism spectrum disorders. Cambridge (MA): Academic Press; 2006. p. 267–84.

59. Kakooza-Mwesige A, Wachtel L, Dhossche D. Catatonia in autism: implications across the life span. Eur Child Adolesc Psychiatry 2008;17(6):327–35.

60. Wachtel L. Treatment of catatonia in autism spectrum disorders. Acta Psychiatr Scand 2019;139:46–55.

61. Bush G, Fink M, Petrides G, et al. Catatonia. II. Treatment with lorazepam and electroconvulsive therapy. Acta Psychiatr Scand 1996;93(2):137–43.

62. McCall W, Shelp F, McDonald W. Controlled investigation of the amobarbital interview in catatonic mutism. Am J Psychiatry 1992;149:202–6.

63. Haq A, Ghaziuddin N. Maintenance electroconvulsive therapy for aggression and self-injurious behavior in two adolescents with autism and catatonia. J Neuropsychiatry Clin Neurosci 2014;26(1):64–72.

64. Ghaziuddin N, Kutcher SP, Knapp P, American Academy of Child and Adolescent Psychiatry Work Group on Quality Issues. Summary of the practice parameter for the use of electroconvulsive therapy with adolescents. J Am Acad Child Adolesc Psychiatry 2004;43(1):119–22.

65. Walter G, Koster K, Rey JM. Electroconvulsive therapy in adolescents: experience, knowledge, and attitudes of recipients. J Am Acad Child Adolesc Psychiatry 1999;38(5):594–9.

66. Ghaziuddin N, Kaza M, Ghazi N, et al. Electroconvulsive therapy for minors: experiences and attitudes of child psychiatrists and psychologists. J ECT 2001; 17(2):109.

67. De Meulenaere M, De Meulenaere J, Ghaziuddin N, et al. Experience, knowledge and attitudes of child and adolescent psychiatrists in Belgium towards pediatric ECT. J ECT 2018;34(4):247–52.

68. Mitchell S, Hassan E, Ghaziuddin N. A follow-up study of electroconvulsive therapy in children and adolescents. J ECT 2018;34(1):40–4.

69. Gelenberg AJ, Mandel MR. Catatonic reaction to high potency neuroleptic drugs. Arch Gen Psychiatry 1977;34:947–50.

70. Ghaziuddin N, Barbosa V, Maixner DF, et al. Catatonia with onset in purberty: ECT response in 2 adolescents. J ECT 2010;26(4):270–6.

71. Cornic F, Consoli A, Tanguy M-L, et al. Association of adolescent catatonia with increased mortality and morbidity: evidence from a prospective follow-up study. Schizophr Res 2009;113(2–3):233–40.

72. Penland HR, Weder N, Tampi RR. The catatonic dilemma expanded. Ann Gen Psychiatry 2006;5(14):x_xx.

73. Levenson JL, Pandurangi AK. Prognosis and complications. In: Caroff SN, Mann SC, Francis A, et al, editors. Catatonia: from psychopathology to neurobiology. Washington, DC: American Psychiatric Publishing; 2004. p. 161–72.

74. Stauder K. Die todliche. Archiv für Psychiatrie und Nervenkrankheiten 1934;102: 614–34.

75. Kraines SH. Bell's Mania. Available at: https://doi.org/10.1176/ajp.91.1.29. Accessed April 29, 2020.

Use of Electroconvulsive Therapy in Autism

Sa Eun Park, MD[a],*, Marco Grados, MD, MPH[b], Lee Wachtel, MD[c], Sanjay Kaji, MD[d]

KEYWORDS

- Autism • Electroconvulsive therapy • Catatonia • Neuroplasticity

KEY POINTS

- The mechanism of action of electroconvulsive therapy (ECT) is not fully elucidated, with prevailing theories ranging from neuroendocrinological to neuroplasticity effects of ECT or epileptiform brain plasticity.
- Youth with autism can present with catatonia as, first described by Wing and Shah, a syndrome that is both similar and different than Kahlbaum's original description.
- ECT is a treatment that can safely and rapidly resolve catatonia in autism and should be considered promptly.
- The literature available for ECT use in youth with autism is consistently growing.
- Under-recognition of the catatonic syndrome and delayed diagnosis and implementation of the anticatatonic treatment paradigms, including ECT, as well as stigma and lack of knowledge of ECT remain clinical stumbling blocks.

INTRODUCTION

After electroconvulsive therapy (ECT) was introduced in 1938 by Cerletti and Bini,[1] the first published case of ECT in youth was in a 3-year-old child with epilepsy.[2] A subsequent case report documented a favorable outcome in 2 adolescents in occupied France in 1942,[3] whereas a case series was published the next year. In 1941, Bender published a case series of youth from Bellevue Hospital who derived benefit from ECT for a variety of affective and psychotic diagnoses and reported no adverse effects. In the next quarter century, close to 400 cases of ECT in youth were reported in the

This article originally appeared in *Child and Adolescent Psychiatric Clinics*, Volume 29, Issue 3, July 2020.

The authors have nothing to disclose. Dr M. Grados received a research contract with Palo Alto Health Sciences, Inc.

[a] Kennedy Krieger Institute, 1741 Ashland Avenue, Baltimore, MD 21205, USA; [b] Johns Hopkins University School of Medicine, 733 North Broadway, Baltimore, MD 21205, USA; [c] Kennedy Krieger Institute, Johns Hopkins School of Medicine, 707 North Broadway Street, Baltimore, MD 21209, USA; [d] Johns Hopkins Hospital, 1800 Orleans Street, Baltimore, MD 21287, USA
* Corresponding author.
E-mail address: Spark172@jhmi.edu

literature,[4] demonstrating a higher acceptance of this procedure by clinicians and families in youth with mental illness. Concerns with risks and side effects associated with ECT, however, generally limited its use to youth who were not developmentally disabled. Early reports of catatonic clinical presentations in youth with autism[5,6] led to attempts to provide ECT to these children.[7] Two landmark studies of catatonia in autism in the early 2000s[8,9] led to accumulating evidence of the prevalence of catatonic features in autism and more extensive consideration for the use of ECT in youth with autism and catatonia.[10] Beyond catatonia, the use of ECT for the treatment of refractory self-injurious behaviors (SIBs) in youth with autism also has gained currency.[11] In this focused review, the clinical presentation, indications, and treatment approaches for the use of ECT in youth with autism are addressed, with an emphasis on catatonia, SIBs, and other conditions for which ECT may be of benefit.

ELECTROCONVULSIVE THERAPY IN THE TREATMENT OF CATATONIA IN AUTISM
Kahlbaum's Catatonia

Moving beyond Griesinger's concept of "unitary psychosis," Kahlbaum and others sought to generate greater diagnostic specificity in relation to psychotic states. In 1874, Kahlbaum's classic "Catatonia or Muscular Tension Insanity" provided a detailed description of a cyclical "muscular disorder" characterized longitudinally by "melancholy, mania, stupor, confusion and later dementia."[12] Kahlbaum describes a first phase of mood changes, followed by a stage of "strange, fixed positions" or "grotesque stereotyped movements…frequent grimacing." Negativism can be present, with resistance of limbs to passive movements. In the later stage of catatonia, a waxy flexibility of limbs is present, which is "unique to the illness." Phases of catatonic excitement can be present; 1 case described "wild, insane behavior, with arbitrary striking, shouting…and biting." In Kahlbaum's description, although thought abnormalities are present, positive symptoms of psychosis are not common (delusions in 5/25 and hallucinations 8/25).[13] Historically, catatonia was considered a sign of worsening schizophrenic illness in both Kraepelin's[14] and Bleuler typologies,[15] a paradigm that was influential well into the 1950s as depicted in Mayer-Gross and colleagues' influential textbook of psychiatry.[16] The automatic association of catatonia with schizophrenia, however, was an error of history. Current understanding of catatonia is that of an independent neurobiological syndrome that has myriad psychiatric, neurologic, medical, and drug-related etiologies. The most common etiology of catatonia is an affective illness, although it took more than a century to sever the previously mandatory link between catatonia and schizophrenia.[17]

Pathophysiology of Catatonia and the Role of Electroconvulsive Therapy

The mechanism of action of ECT is not fully elucidated,[18] with long-standing theories revolving around neuroendocrinological changes and newer theories based on neuroplasticity effects of ECT or epileptiform brain plasticity.[19] These effects include axonal sprouting and synaptic reorganizations,[20] hippocampal mossy fiber sprouting,[21] hippocampal dentate gyrus neurogenesis,[22] neurotrophic growth factor induction 2,[23] generation of calretinin-positive interneurons,[24] and NARP-mediated enhanced dendritic arborization[25] among others. Although ECT, a form of controlled seizures, can induce beneficial effects on neuronal systems, clinical seizures per se can cause neuronal damage,[26] such as a reduction in newly born hippocampal granule cells in juvenile seizures[27] and necrotic damage of the thalamus in status epilepticus.[28] Clinical seizures in an uncontrolled setting also are, of course, associated with risks that are mitigated in modern convulsive therapy under anesthesia with full neuromuscular blockade and ongoing oxygenation. In models of epilepsy, a decrease in GABAergic interneurons is prominent,[29] most critical for inhibitory interneuron chandelier cells.[30] The loss of parvalbumin-interneurons in other models of epilepsy parallels the severity of seizures, leads to kindling phenomena, and increases the clinical severity of epilepsy.[31] Admittedly, the decrease of interneurons in epileptic foci contrasts with the increase in interneurons reported after ECT-triggered neurogenesis.[24]

Identifiable structural brain differences are not uniformly found in patients with catatonia; rather, various organic brain abnormalities appear to result in a final common pathway. In a review of 57 patients with catatonia, more than one-third had an identifiable difference in brain scans; however, the nature of these were variable, including periventricular changes (8/22) and ischemic gliosis (3/22).[32] Frontotemporal lobe atrophy symptoms overlap with catatonia, and a case series documents catatonic conditions in 3 patients with frontotemporal dementia (FTD).[33] Earlier reports had identified cerebellar atrophy[34] as well as brainstem and vermis atrophy[35] in patients with catatonia. In addition, catatonia may be a complication of autoimmune and infectious processes, including encephalitis lethargica or limbic encephalitis,[36] systemic lupus erythematosus,[37] and anti-NMDA receptor encephalitis.[38] Finally, catatonic states as a traumatic withdrawal syndrome in asylum-seeking children in Scandinavian countries also has been reported as a "giving up syndrome," perhaps akin to historical descriptions of catatonic states amongst displaced persons after World War II and other crises of humanity.[39] In summary, catatonic states can occur through multiple pathways and result in phenotypically similar states with overlapping symptoms while having varying etiologies. The catatonic syndrome originally described by Kahlbaum may be a more specific condition within a catatonic spectrum of conditions that manifests primarily in severely mentally ill patients with affective and/or psychotic disorders but also is readily seen across multiple other somatic medical conditions and unfortunately often not detected in a timely fashion.

Clinical Features of Catatonia in Autism

Catatonic symptoms are estimated to be prevalent at a rate of up to 12% to 17% in adolescents and young adults with autism[40] and require a high degree of clinical suspicion for proper identification. Structured approaches to the assessment of catatonia are not widely disseminated. The Bush-Francis Catatonia Rating Scale (BFCRS) (1996) is widely used in clinical practice and research for the evaluation of catatonia. Individuals with autism and catatonia, however, preferentially express echophenomena, stereotypy, mannerisms, rituals, mutism, negativism, and repetitive psychomotor behaviors, which are not as well elicited by the BFCRS. It also is salient that some of these symptoms overlap with the core symptoms of autism that may have been present for years, and appropriate evaluation of symptoms that are a departure from the youth's baseline are essential. In 2006, diagnostic criteria specific for catatonia in autism were proposed, in which mutism was replaced with drastically decreased speech and the duration of symptoms noted to be longer.[41] The suggested criteria include (1) immobility, drastically decreased speech, or stupor of at least 1-day duration, associated with at least 1 of the following: catalepsy, automatic obedience, or posturing, and (2) in the absence of immobility, drastically decreased speech, or stupor, a marked worsening from baseline is present for at least 1 week in at least 1 of the following: slowness of movement or speech, difficulty in initiating movements or speech unless prompted, freezing during actions, difficulty crossing lines, inability to cease actions, stereotypy, echophenomena, catalepsy, automatic obedience, posturing, negativism, or ambitendency (ie, patient appears motorically stuck in indecisive hesitant movement). A medical work-up to rule out organic causes should include (1) complete medical history; (2) physical and neurologic examination; (3) laboratory work directed at immune, genetic, and developmental disorders; (4) imaging, including computed tomography or magnetic resonance imaging, to rule out structural brain abnormalities in those presenting with focal neurologic signs; (5) toxicology tests to rule out substance-induced symptoms; and (6) electroencephalogram when clinically indicated and there is a suspicion of seizure disorder.

Although the differential diagnosis of catatonia in autism is broad, and organic causes always should be suspected and explored, the role of obsessional slowness merits scrutiny. Obsessional slowness is a state of slowed motor purposeful movements seen in individuals with obsessive-compulsive disorder (OCD) and/or autism. It is a chronic, progressive condition, which may be resistant to usual treatment.[42] In 1 series of patients with OCD, up to 28% showed some degree of obsessional slowness, including slowly performing common daily tasks not associated with psychotic or affective symptoms. In more extreme cases, daily tasks can take up to hours and cause severe impairment, such as malnutrition, dehydration, and inability to complete necessary activities of daily living.[43] The diagnostic differential is critical, because obsessional slowness responds preferentially to behavior therapy and serotonin-augmenting agents,[44] whereas some instances of obsessional slowness may overlap with catatonia in patients on the autism spectrum and treatment approaches to catatonia may be merited.[45,46]

In summary, catatonia should be considered in individuals with autism after a change in baseline function in areas of psychomotor activity, activities of daily living, functional skills (such as speech), behavioral activities, appetite, and sleep, including symptoms in **Box 1**. Taking a detailed history of baseline level of functioning is critical when there is suspicion of emerging catatonia.

Case Presentation

A 17-year-old girl with a past psychiatric history of autism spectrum disorder, intellectual disability, and cyclical mood disorder was admitted to the inpatient psychiatric

---

Box 1
Clinical manifestations of catatonia in autism

Catatonia symptoms
  Odd gait
  Freezing
  Stiff postures
  Slowness
  Needing frequent prompting
  Hesitation to initiate movement (eg, crossing thresholds, moving from sitting to standing)
  Changes in sleep pattern
  Hyperactivity and impulsiveness
  Stereotypy
  Negativism (opposition or no response to instructions or external stimuli)
  Difficulty stopping actions
  Bizarre thoughts and psychosis
  Decrease in speech or development of mutism
  Incontinence

Data from Wing L, Shah A. Catatonia in autistic spectrum disorders. Br J Psychiatry 2000;176:357-62; and Wachtel LE, Shorter E, Fink M. Electroconvulsive therapy for self-injurious behaviour in autism spectrum disorders: Recognizing catatonia is key. Curr Opin Psychiatry 2018;31(2):116-122.

unit for worsening manic symptoms, including heightened irritability, insomnia, pressured speech, racing thoughts, and distractibility. She also was increasingly impulsive, hyperverbal, and disorganized. Outpatient medications included olanzapine, 20 mg; lithium, 1500 mg, for mood stabilization; and clonazepam, 1 mg, for anxiety. During inpatient admission, olanzapine was switched to fluphenazine, which helped stabilize manic symptoms. As the manic symptoms began to improve, however, the patient began to have episodic waxy flexibility, posturing, cogwheeling, echopraxia, and mumbling. She would hold a specific position for minutes and could not be redirected. She had difficulty eating and drinking and could not perform activities of daily living. These symptoms were assessed to correspond to catatonia. Clonazepam was switched to lorazepam to target catatonic symptoms. Lorazepam was increased to 8 mg daily with limited further improvement. The patient continued to have episodes of slowed movements and randomly "getting stuck." Due to minimal improvement of catatonia, ECT was instituted, including 12 ECT treatments and 12 maintenance-ECT (m-ECT) sessions. Toward the end of the ECT regimen, the patient performing her own ADLs, was more alert to her surroundings and staff, more responsive and interactive, and motorically more flexible. Additionally, she was able to eat by herself and her speech was more intelligible. The family also reported that she was closer to baseline compared with her status at admission. The patient's genetic profile included a prior finding of loss of the gene *MMACHC* function and premutation fragile X triplet repeats. Variants in the recessive gene, methylmalonic aciduria, and homocystinuria type C protein (*MMACHC*) are associated with methylmalonic acidemia with homocystinuria. The human phenotype ontology for *MMACHC* includes abnormality of extrapyramidal motor function, anorexia, cerebral cortical atrophy, and cystathioninemia, all of which may have overlapping symptoms with catatonia and manifest in later years.

Electroconvulsive Therapy Treatment of Catatonia in Autism

According to Leonhard's nosology of catatonia, 2 essentially different forms of catatonia can be distinguished, namely periodic catatonia (with an acute onset, shows an intermittent course with incomplete remission) and the group of systematic catatonia (with an insidious onset, shows a chronic and progressive course without remission).[47] Although gradual onset is more common, a sudden onset of catatonia has been associated with higher rates of remission.[48] Overall, early recognition and adequate, prompt treatment are needed for a favorable prognosis.[49] Effective treatment includes stress reduction and structure in mild instances and use of lorazepam and/or ECT in established catatonia[41]

   Benzodiazepines are used as an initial approach to the treatment of catatonia in autism due to their rapid onset of action to ameliorate symptoms, their potential utility in forming a diagnostic impression, and their potential use as the sole treatment of some patients with catatonia. The most effective benzodiazepine is lorazepam, which like all benzodiazepines is a GABA-A receptor agonist. Lorazepam is favored due to its rapid onset (1–3 minutes intravenously [IV]), its safe side effect profile, and its status as Food and Drug Administration–approved for anxiety, insomnia, and preanesthesia.[50] An initial dose of lorazepam, 1 mg to 2 mg, used either sublingually, IV, or intramuscularly—if the oral route is not available—can be given as a challenge dose, repeated every 3 hours to 4 hours, with increasing dosing up to 4 mg/d to 8 mg/d initially. In some case series, upwards of 80% of patients respond to the challenge. For younger patients, a lower dose of lorazepam may be more appropriate, with eventual titration as indicated clinically.[51] If a patient responds to lorazepam, it may be continued with titration to 12 mg/d to 16 mg/d as tolerated, although there are reports of patients requiring higher dosages of benzodiazepines for sustained catatonia remission. Close clinical monitoring is essential, because lorazepam response may require increasing dose to manage symptoms and its efficacy may decline over time. If response to lorazepam is not substantial or sustained, ECT should be considered. Zolpidem has been linked to improvement in select patients with catatonia and FTD and often is used as a challenge test for the catatonia diagnosis in European settings.[52]

ECT, in particular bilateral ECT, is a definitive treatment of catatonia in autism due to its high response rate when the diagnosis is ascertained correctly. ECT should be considered when high-dose lorazepam does not result in effective relief of symptoms or when autonomic dysfunction occurs. Autonomic changes in catatonia, including hemodynamic and thermoregulatory instability, as well as softer signs of acrocyanosis, flushing, and profuse diaphoresis, herald the onset of malignant catatonia. Initially described in 1934 by Stauder, malignant catatonia has a 10% to 20% fatality rate if untreated, and immediate implementation of ECT is recommended. In 2004, the American Academy of Child & Adolescent Psychiatry (AACAP) published practice parameters for the use of ECT in minors. In these criteria, patients must have (1) a diagnosis of severe major depressive disorder, mania, schizoaffective disorder, schizophrenia, catatonia, or neuroleptic malignant syndrome; (2) symptom severity that is persistently disabling or life threatening; and (3) failure to respond to at least 2 adequate trials of appropriate psychopharmacologic agents accompanied by other appropriate treatment modalities.[53] In the guidelines, the suggestion also is made that ECT be considered earlier when (1) adequate medication trials are not possible because of a patient's inability to tolerate psychopharmacologic treatment, (2) the adolescent is grossly incapacitated and thus cannot take medication, or (3) waiting for a response to a psychopharmacologic treatment may endanger the life of the adolescent. It is relevant to emphasize that the AACAP guidelines require 2 failed psychotropic trials and not exhaustion of the entire US pharmacy before ECT is pursued.

Full ascertainment of the diagnosis of catatonia in autism is key. Baseline symptoms of autism may overlap with mild catatonic symptoms, which may delay diagnosis. Therefore, patients with autism and catatonia may receive treatment only at later stages of the illness, when more severe symptoms are present, leading to severe debilitation and gross incapacitation. The importance of identifying the catatonic syndromic presentation in autism is critical because it may represent a distinct subtype with a particularly poor outcome.[54] An increasing number of case reports demonstrate a swift and effective response of catatonia in autism to ECT. A recent report documented the treatment course of 22 predominantly male youth with autism ages, 6 years to 26 years, diagnosed with catatonia. All patients received ECT after a trial of lorazepam, 1 mg to 27 mg daily, with ECT sessions ranging from 16 to 688. Alleviation of catatonia with SIBs using ECT was noted in this cohort. The data also suggest that for patients who require ECT, m-ECT often becomes indefinitely imperative, with m-ECT frequencies as often as weekly to sustain symptom remission. Akin to many modern pharmacotherapeutics, ECT is a treatment, not a cure, and m-ECT needs to be sustained over long periods of time.[55]

As in the adult population, efficacy of ECT in youth may be affected by several technical factors, including but not limited to electrode placement, frequency of ECT, and the quality of seizure elicited. Regarding the placement of electrodes in ECT, in general, unilateral placement has been preferred when treating major depression due to reported decreased cognitive side effects.[56] Bilateral placement is favored when a more rapid-onset therapeutic effect is needed and is the recommended electrode placement for the treatment of catatonia.[57] Unlike unilateral ECT, which requires doses of 8-times to 12-times initial seizure threshold for a therapeutic seizure, bilateral ECT doses range from 0.5-times to 1.5-times initial seizure threshold. These doses may be fully effective, with maximal recommended doses in the range of 2.5-times seizure threshold.[58] For the best therapeutic response, a robust generalization of the electrically induced seizure of sufficient duration and optimal postictal suppression must occur in the presence of adequate hydration, sufficient hyperventilation, use of flumazenil to counteract benzodiazepine effects, and consistent monitoring. The likelihood of developing a transient delirium during an ECT series is greater, however, with bilateral electrode placement.

Per the 2004 AACAP guidelines, ECT may begin at either 2 times or 3 times weekly, with changes to the schedule if significant cognitive side effects arise. The treatment course of ECT typically is categorized into acute ECT and m-ECT phases, wherein the acute treatment course typically is up to 12 sessions at 3 times per week, whereas the m-ECT course at lesser frequency is to prevent symptom relapse. There are no empirical data, however, to support an ideal number of treatments for catatonia in autism. In a retrospective review of 22 autistic patients diagnosed with catatonia over a 12-year period, all patients received acute ECT and m-ECT, with more than 50% of the cohort having received more than 100 treatments during the study period.[55]

ELECTROCONVULSIVE THERAPY IN THE TREATMENT OF SELF-INJURIOUS BEHAVIORS AND AGGRESSION IN AUTISM

In autism, SIB manifests as repetitive motor patterns with typical topographies causing bodily damage. SIBs in autism may occur in the spectrum of repetitive movements (stereotypies) or in response to operant or environmental, functions. The latter presentation is readily addressed with applied behavioral analysis strategies involving delineation of specific social functions to the behavior and associated behavioral treatments. Some SIBs are devoid of operant function, however, and the high-frequency nature of the damaging acts singles them out as a particularly malignant form of repetitive behavior. Topographies of SIB reported by caregivers of children with autism include repetitive self-directed actions of biting, hitting, punching body parts; head or limb banging; pulling of body appendages or hair; and poking of sensitive body parts. Varying degrees of SIBs are present not only in individuals with autism, with higher rates associated with cognitive and communication impairments and psychiatric and medical comorbidities, but also in those living in restricted settings. The consequences of SIB can range from minor to severe, such as fractures, infections, disfigurement, loss of vision or hearing, and intracranial damage. SIBs can cause interpersonal problems, leading to poor social relationships, difficulty with caregiving of such individuals, and higher risk of out-of-home placement more restrictive settings.

SIBs in autism can be conceptualized as part of the catatonia spectrum, because a stereotypy common to both catatonia and autism.[11] In a literature review on the use of ECT for individuals with autism and severe SIB encompassing 1982 to 2008, 11 reports were identified. Favorable evidence was present for marked benefit of ECT used for intractable, repetitive SIB. ECT parameters included (1) continuous oxygenation through face mask, sedation with propofol or methohexital, muscle relaxation with succinylcholine, and, for those treated with benzodiazepines, the administration of flumazenil; (2) bitemporal electrode placement; (3) initial stimulation energy based on half-age formula, with subsequent energy dosing to assure effective seizures; and (4) acute treatment course of thrice weekly treatments until SIB incidence decreases or plateaus.[59]

It is important to recognize that repetitive self-injury in autism often is associated with other catatonic symptoms; thus, a thorough assessment of catatonia should be conducted. Multiple case reports in recent years have documented the successful treatment of intractable SIB in autistic youth who concomitantly demonstrated other catatonic symptomology as well as comorbid psychotic and/or affective diagnoses. Given that individuals with autism and intellectual disability have higher rates of psychopathology than those who are neurotypical, it may be the case that catatonia in autism often is fueled by both the underlying autistic substrate as well as additional psychiatric illness rendered more likely in the autistic brain.

ELECTROCONVULSIVE THERAPY IN THE TREATMENT OF MAJOR DEPRESSION, BIPOLAR DISORDER, AND SCHIZOPHRENIA IN AUTISM

A diagnosis of severe comorbid psychiatric disorders in autism is a challenge that clinicians face due to the lack of standardized assessment tools for comorbid psychiatric disorder in autism and intellectual disability despite the increasing recognition of comorbid conditions. It is well recognized that comorbid psychiatric conditions in autism are common, with studies focused on the emergence and characteristics of comorbid conditions in autism, but there are few data available to guide diagnosis and treatment of severe psychiatric illness in autism. Although in neurotypical children ECT has been used in severe mood disorders[60] and schizophrenia spectrum disorders,[61] there are no current data on its use in these disorders in autism, except in the cases, discussed previously, where affective and psychotic illness was present with catatonia.

SUMMARY AND FUTURE DIRECTIONS

ECT is indicated for catatonia in autism given the high rate of therapeutic response documented in multiple case series in the literature. The field does not yet benefit from controlled clinical trials, however, which are made difficult due to ethical concerns, difficulty in accumulating cases, and lack of interest from industry.[46] The often dire clinical status of catatonic autistic youth also makes classic research studies challenging, because these patients require rapid treatment to avoid severe clinical consequence, bodily injury, or even death. Notwithstanding, increased education to providers on the identification of catatonic states in individuals with autism is a crucial first step in delivering safe and effective ECT treatment, which has a high rate of benefiting such difficult to treat conditions in a vulnerable population.

REFERENCES

1. Cerletti U, Bini L. Un nuovo metodo di shockterapie:'l'elettroshock'(riassunto). Reale Accademia Medica; 1938. Communicazione alla seduta del 28 maggio 1938-XVI della Reale Accademia Medica di Roma.
2. Hemphill RE, Walter. The treatment of mental disorders by electrically induced convulsions. J Ment Sci 1941;87(367):256–75.
3. Heuyer G, Bour LR, Leroy R. L'electrochoc chez les enfants. Ann Med Psychol (Paris) 1943;2:402–7.
4. Rey JM, Walter G. Half a century of ECT use in young people. Am J Psychiatry 1997;154(5):595–602.
5. Realmuto GM. Catatonia in autistic disorder: a sign of comorbidity or variable expression? J Autism Dev Disord 1991;21(4):517–28.
6. Dhossche D. Brief report: catatonia in autistic disorders. J Autism Dev Disord 1998;28(4):329–31.
7. Brasic JR, Zagzag D. Progressive catatonia. Psychol Rep 1999;84(1):239–46.
8. Wing L, Shah A. Catatonia in autistic spectrum disorders. Br J Psychiatry 2000; 176:357–62.

9. Wing L, Shah A. A systematic examination of catatonia-like clinical pictures in autism spectrum disorders. Int Rev Neurobiol 2006;72:21–39.

10. Dhossche DM. Autism as early expression of catatonia. Med Sci Monit 2004; 10(3). RA31–R39.

11. Wachtel LE, Dhossche DM. Self-injury in autism as an alternate sign of catatonia: implications for electroconvulsive therapy. Med Hypotheses 2010;75(1):111–4.

12. Kahlbaum KL. Catatonia: translated from the German Die Katatonie oder das Spannungsirresein. In: Levij Y, Pridan T, editors. Baltimore (MD): The Johns Hopkins University Press; 1973.

13. Kendler KS. The development of kraepelin's mature diagnostic concept of catatonic dementia praecox: a close reading of relevant texts. Schizophr Bull 2019. https://doi.org/10.1093/schbul/sbz101.

14. Gazdag G, Takacs R, Ungvari GS. Catatonia as a putative nosological entity: a historical sketch. World J Psychiatry 2017;7(3):177–83.

15. Rogers D. Catatonia: a contemporary approach. J Neuropsychiatry Clin Neurosci 1991;3(3):334–40.

16. Mayer-Gross W, Slater E, Roth M. Clinical psychiatry. 2nd edition. Williams and Wilkins; 1960.

17. Fink M, Shorter E, Taylor MA. Catatonia is not schizophrenia: Kraeplin's error and the need to recognize catatonia as an independent syndrome in medical nomenclature. Schizophr Bull 2010;36(2):314–20.

18. Singh A, Kar SK. How electroconvulsive therapy works?: understanding the neurobiological mechanisms. Clin Psychopharmacol Neurosci 2017;15(3): 210–21.

19. Scott BW, Wang S. Kindling-induced neurogenesis in the dentate gyrus of the rat. Neurosci Lett 1998;248(2):73–6.

20. Sutula T, He XX. Synaptic reorganization in the hippocampus induced by abnormal functional activity. Science 1988;239(4844):1147–50.

21. Gombos Z, Spiller A, Cottrell GA, et al. Mossy fiber sprouting induced by repeated electroconvulsive shock seizures. Brain Res 1999;844(1–2):28–33.

22. Scott BW, Wojtowicz JM, Burnham WM, et al. Neurogenetics in the dentate gyrus of the rat following electroconvulsive shock seizures. Exp Neurol 2000;165(2): 231–6.

23. Kondratyev A, Ved R, Gale K, et al. The effects of repeated minimal electroconvulsive shock exposure on levels of mRNA encoding fibroblast growth factor-2 and nerve growth factor in limbic regions. Neuroscience 2002;114(2):411–6.

24. Inta D, Lima-Ojeda JM, Lau T, et al. Electroconvulsive therapy induces neurogenesis in frontal rat brain areas. PLoS One 2013;8(7):e69869.

25. Chang AD, Vaidya PV, Retzbach EP, et al. Narp mediates antidepressant-like effects of electroconvulsive seizures. Neuropsychopharmacology 2018;43(5): 1088–98.

26. Homes GL. Seizure-induced neuronal injury: animal data. Neurology 2002;59(9 Suppl 5):S3–6.

27. McCabe BK, Silveira DC, Cilio MR, et al. Reduced neurogenesis after neonatal seizures. J Neurosci 2001;21(6):2094–103.

28. Druga R, Mares P, Otáhal J, et al. Degenerative neuronal changes in the rat thalamus induced by status epilepticus at different developmental stages. Epilepsy Res 2005;63(1):43–65.

29. Ribak CE, Harris AB, Vaughn JE, et al. Inhibitory, GABAergic nerve terminals decrease at sites of focal epilepsy. Science 1979;205(4402):211–4.

30. DeFelipe J. Chandelier cells and epilepsy. Brain 1999;122(Pt 10):1807–22.

31. van Vliet EA, Aronica E, Tolner EA, et al. Progression of temporal lobe epilepsy in the rat is associated with immunocytochemical changes in inhibitory interneurons in specific regions of the hippocampal formation. Exp Neurol 2004;187(2): 367-79.

32. Unal A, Altindag A, Demir B, et al. The use of lorazepam and electroconvulsive therapy in the treatment of catatonia: treatment characteristics and outcomes in 60 patients. J ECT 2017;33(4):290-3.

33. Utumi Y, Iseki E, Arai H. Three patients with mood disorders showing catatonia and frontotemporal lobes atrophy. Psychogeriatrics 2013;13(4):254-9.

34. Wilcox JA. Cerebellar atrophy and catatonia. Biol Psychiatry 1991;29(7):733-4.

35. Joseph AB, Anderson WH, O'Leary DH, et al. Brainstem and vermis atrophy in catatonia. Am J Psychiatry 1985;142(3):352-4.

36. Ali S, Welch CA, Park LT, et al. Encephalitis and catatonia treated with ECT. Cogn Behav Neurol 2008;21(1):46-51.

37. Boeke A, Pullen B, Coppes L, et al. Catatonia associated with systemic lupus erythematosus (SLE): a report of two cases and a review of the literature. Psychosomatics 2018;59(6):523-30.

38. Espinola-Nadurille M, Flores-Rivera J, Rivas-Alonso V, et al. Catatonia in patients with anti-NMDA receptor encephalitis. Psychiatry Clin Neurosci 2019;73(9): 574-80.

39. von Knorring AL, Hultcrantz E. Asylum-seeking children with resignation syndrome: catatonia or traumatic withdrawal syndrome? Eur Child Adolesc Psychiatry 2019. https://doi.org/10.1007/s00787-019-01427-0.

40. Withane N, Dhossche DM. Electroconvulsive treatment for catatonia in autism spectrum disorders. Child Adolesc Psychiatr Clin N Am 2019;28(1):101-10.

41. Dhossche DM, Shah A, Wing L. Blueprints for the assessment, treatment, and future study of catatonia in autism spectrum disorders. Int Rev Neurobiol 2006; 72:267-84.

42. Ganos C, Kassavetis P, Cerdan M, et al. Revisiting the syndrome of "obsessional slowness". Mov Disord Clin Pract 2015;2(2):163-9.

43. Hymas N, Lees A, Bolton D, et al. The neurology of obsessional slowness. Brain 1991;114(Pt 5):2203-33.

44. Singh G, Sharan P, Grover S, et al. Obsessive slowness: a case report. Indian J Psychiatry 2003;45(1):60-1.

45. Dos Santos-Ribeiro S, de Salles Andrade JB, Quintas JN, et al. A systematic review of the utility of electroconvulsive therapy in broadly defined obsessive-compulsive-related disorders. Prim Care Companion CNS Disord 2018;20(5). https://doi.org/10.4088/PCC.18r02342.

46. Kellner CH, Wachtel LE, Dhossche D. Electroconvulsive therapy is helpful for patients with obsessive-compulsive disorder-related disorders: a response to dos santos-ribeiro et al. Prim Care Companion CNS Disord 2019;21(3). https://doi.org/10.4088/PCC.18l02414.

47. Pfuhlman B, Stober G. The different conceptions of catatonia: historical overview and critical discussion. Eur Arch Psychiatry Clin Neurosci 2001;251(Suppl 1):I4-7.

48. Ohta M, Kano Y, Nagai Y, et al. Catatonia in individuals with autism spectrum disorders in adolescence and early adulthood: a long-term prospective study. Int Rev Neurobiol 2006;72:41-54.

49. Taylor MA, Fink M. Catatonia in psychiatric classification: a home of its own. Am J Psychiatry 2003;160(7):1233-41.

50. Ghiasi N, Bhansali RK, Marwaha R. Lorazepam. In: StatPearls. Treasure Island (FL): StatPearls Publishing LLC; 2020. NBK532890.
51. Rasmussen SA, Mazurek MF, Rosebush PI. Catatonia: our current understanding of its diagnosis, treatment and pathophysiology. World J Psychiatry 2016;6(4): 391–8.
52. Isomura S, Monji A, Sasaki K, et al. FTD with catatonia-like signs that temporarily resolved with zolpidem. Neurol Clin Pract 2013;3(4):354–7.
53. Ghaziuddin N, Kutcher SP, Knapp P, et al. Practice parameter for use of electroconvulsive therapy with adolescents. J Am Acad Child Adolesc Psychiatry 2004; 43(12):1521–39.
54. Ghaziuddin M, Quinlan P, Ghaziuddin N, et al. Catatonia in autism: a distinct subtype? J Intellect Disabil Res 2005;49(Pt 1):102–5.
55. Wachtel LE. Treatment of catatonia in autism spectrum disorders. Acta Psychiatr Scand 2019;139(1):46–55.
56. Kellner CH, Knapp R, Husain MM, et al. Bifrontal, bitemporal and right unilateral electrode placement in ECT: randomised trial. Br J Psychiatry 2010;196(3): 226–34.
57. Kellner CH, McCall WV. The FDA final order on ECT devices, Finally. J ECT 2019; 35(2):69–70.
58. Greenberg RM, Kellner CH. Electroconvulsive therapy: a selected review. Am J Geriatr Psychiatry 2005;13(4):268–81.
59. Wachtel LE, Shorter E, Fink M, et al. Electroconvulsive therapy for self-injurious behaviour in autism spectrum disorders: recognizing catatonia is key. Curr Opin Psychiatry 2018;31(2):116–22.
60. Walter G, Rey JM. An epidemiological study of the use of ECT in adolescents. J Am Acad Child Adolesc Psychiatry 1997;36(6):809–15.
61. Baeza I, Flamarique I, Garrido JM, et al. Clinical experience using electroconvulsive therapy in adolescents with schizophrenia spectrum disorders. J Child Adolesc Psychopharmacol 2010;20(3):205–9.

Autism Spectrum Disorder and Substance Use Disorder
A Dual Diagnosis Hiding in Plain Sight

Elizabeth Kunreuther, MSW, LCSW, LCAS*

KEYWORDS

- Autism spectrum disorder • Substance use disorder • Prevention • Treatment
- Constructed narrative • Cognitive dissonance

KEY POINTS

- Individuals diagnosed with autism spectrum disorder (ASD) have double the risk of developing a substance use disorder (SUD) compared with the general population.
- Many factors can contribute to the development of co-occurring ASD and SUD. However, the research and literature addressing this particular comorbidity is scarce.
- Evidence-informed prevention, screening, and treatment approaches are possible when providers from both the ASD and SUD communities collaborate to adapt protocols.
- Constructed narratives associated with both disorders may be at the root of the scientific and medical communities' disinterest in this life-threatening comorbidity.
- Clinicians should always screen for SUD in cognitively able individuals with ASD and, if present, develop appropriate treatment plans to address the comorbidity.

INTRODUCTION

Substance use disorders (SUDs) are a problem for adolescents and young adults with autism spectrum disorder (ASD). A quantitative study drawn from Swedish registry data showed that individuals diagnosed with autism spectrum disorder (ASD) have double the risk of developing an SUD compared with the non-ASD control group.[1] This finding is in contrast with the prevailing wisdom that SUDs are not as common in ASD, possibly because of ASD providing protective factors for the comorbidity.[2] Therefore, screening individuals with autism for SUD is not the general practice. There is a dearth of general epidemiologic research and treatment studies for the population.[3] There is no clinical evidence explaining the lack of attention to the dual diagnosis of ASD and SUD. This disconnect may be understood by considering the distinct

This article originally appeared in Child and Adolescent Psychiatric Clinics, Volume 29, Issue 3, July 2020.

Department of Psychiatry, University of North Carolina School of Medicine, Chapel Hill, NC, USA

* UNC WakeBrook Addiction and Detox Center, 107 Sunnybrook Road, Raleigh, NC 27610.

E-mail address: elizabeth_kunreuther@med.unc.edu

Psychiatr Clin N Am 44 (2021) 35–49
https://doi.org/10.1016/j.psc.2020.11.004
0193-953X/21/© 2020 Elsevier Inc. All rights reserved.

culturally constructed narratives for ASD and SUD: the ASD narrative depicts the individual as innocent and deserving, whereas the narrative of SUD depicts an individual as degenerate and unworthy. Allowing for a relationship between ASD and SUDs also sanctions the intersection of the stereotypes created by their associated narratives, leading to cognitive dissonance. Clinicians should overcome this bias, screen individuals with ASD for SUD, provide appropriate treatment, and conduct research into this prevalent and life-threatening comorbidity. Despite minimal research and literature addressing a dual diagnosis of autism spectrum and substance use diagnoses, there are recommendations for preventive strategies, adapted assessments, and treatment possibilities.

A DUAL DIAGNOSIS: AUTISM SPECTRUM AND SUBSTANCE USE DISORDERS

SUD has been considered rare in individuals with ASD.[1,2] Prior studies have reported rates from 0.7% to 36% and have had significant limitations.[3] Drexel University National Outcomes Indicator Report: Transition to Adulthood's section on high-risk behaviors reports about a third of respondents having at least 1 drink of alcohol and 8% using illicit substances in the past 30 days.[4] No follow-up questions were asked regarding frequency or quantity of consumption. The report's dataset, culled from individuals seeking or mandated to seek special education services, may omit precisely those individuals with ASD most at risk for developing an SUD, those who have been successfully mainstreamed and no longer seek or require special education but still may not fit in. As Clarke and colleagues[5] noted in their study, individuals with ASD used alcohol to help ease social anxiety and to facilitate social interaction. Butwicka and colleagues[1] had a broader dataset, Swedish population registries, to identify a 2-fold higher risk for substance use–related problems in individuals with ASD without attention-deficit/hyperactivity disorder (ADHD) or intellectual disability. ASD with ADHD conferred the highest risk in the sample.

Shared Comorbidities

Although there is scant literature addressing a dual diagnosis of SUD and ASD, a connection between the 2 disorders would make logical sense. Individuals with depression, anxiety, ADHD, and a history of witnessing or experiencing violence (such as being bullied) are at a significantly higher risk for developing an SUD, and individuals with ASD have appreciably higher rates of depression, anxiety, ADHD, and victimization from bullying than the general population.[4,6–8]

Despite limited evidence-based research linking ASD and SUD, it is not difficult to make the connection that people with autism would be at greater risk for developing an SUD because of the well-documented and studied comorbidities associated with both autism and SUDs.

Behavioral Connections

There are other connections between substance use and autism, such as behavioral connections. The author and self-advocate Maia Szalavitz[9] addresses the behavioral associations in her book, *The Unbroken Brain*: "It seems that the same regions that gave me my intense curiosity, obsessive focus, and ability to learn and memorize quickly also made me vulnerable to discovering potential bad habits and then rapidly getting locked into them."[9(p17)] Characteristics of ASD include repetitive, compulsive, obsessive behaviors and special interests. The same could be said for SUD. With autism, the repetitive behaviors manifest themselves in movements such as rocking or stimming, but they can also present as ritualistic behaviors.[10] SUD also has ritualistic elements: addiction to a substance is learned behavior that occurs after administering the substance repetitively. It is repetitive behaviors that can eventually lead to dependence. In addition, like a "special interest" for those with autism, individuals with SUD often report a ritualized aspect to their use, at least initially. There is also evidence that, for individuals with SUD, finding and administering the substance, particularly an illicit substance, is almost as addictive as the substance itself.[11]

Self-Medication

Another connection between ASD and SUD is self-medication. The book *Asperger Syndrome and Alcohol: Drinking to Cope* hypothesizes that it was the coauthor Matthew Tinsley's anxiety and undiagnosed ASD that led to his alcohol misuse.[12] Online, there are hundreds of posts and video testimonials by people with ASD who use substances. The content of these postings suggest that individuals with ASD use alcohol or illicit substances to relieve anxiety, increase social empathy, ease social communication, reduce stress, and dampen sensory stimulation.[13–15] Tinsley and colleagues[12] describe alcohol as a "numbing device which enables tolerance, integration, acceptance and flexibility, which the person with AS [Asperger syndrome] may not naturally possess."[12(p22)]

Tinsley and colleagues,[12] Szalavitz,[9] and many online posters report that substance use is also a means of coping with an undiagnosed/misdiagnosed developmental disorder. Some patients suggest that a lack of a proper diagnosis was the cause of their substance use rather than the traits and comorbidities related to their ASD. However, Butwicka and colleagues'[1] findings, along with anecdotal evidence from online forums, suggest it is not only those undiagnosed/misdiagnosed that self-medicate. Although the evidence is for the most part anecdotal, it is clear that individuals diagnosed early in life may also seek substances to self-medicate uncomfortable aspects of their autism. "I'm a 20 year old guy. Ever since I was about 14 I have used all kinds of drugs (marijuana, Adderall, pain killers) to help me feel better about having this 'disorder'. For a 4 year span I became addicted to pain killers. They make me feel 'normal' and help me forget about being an Aspie."[16]

Acceptance and Fitting in

There is a fundamental factor as to why adolescents with or without autism abuse alcohol and drugs: fitting in.[17] Although awareness of ASD has reduced stigma among the general population, people with ASD often know they are different and many report they struggle with not fitting in. The Centers for Disease Control and Prevention cites bullying, both verbal and physical, as a risk factor for developing an SUD, and, according to the National Outcomes Indicator Report: Transition to Adulthood, half of the individuals surveyed cited they were victims of bullying.[4,18] It should be no surprise that adolescents might start to drink or use drugs to cope or as a means to assimilate with their neurotypical peers. Assimilation requires a wide range of adaptations, including tolerating some of the ritual school activities that promote social bonding, such as sporting events, parties, and dances. People with ASD claim that substances can help them to manage sensory sensitivities that are a part of daily life:

> I did go to a normal high school and I couldn't cope with it. It was too big and I didn't really get on with anyone in my class. I remember being in the corridor when the bell went for another lesson and everyone just came out at once and went to go to their next room and I thought "God, this is absolutely horrific." It [high school] was just really, really overwhelming.[19]

One ASD blogger wrote that in high school the only crowd that would accept him were the people who used marijuana and other illicit substances because they were more tolerant of his differences. "I was friendless through high school, but when I started meeting people who smoked cannabis I found it much easier to make friends with them. Many of them also used psilocybin and LSD, so they were used to being around people with much weirder behavior than mine."[20]

Biological Connections

Various studies seem to indicate biological connections between the 2 diagnoses. There is research addressing genetic connections as well as overlapping neural circuits and molecular signaling pathways in both autism and SUDs. For example, in Butwicka and colleagues[1] study, parents and siblings of individuals with ASD also had an increased risk for developing an SUD. Patrick Rothwell[21] released an article describing a host of neurologic similarities between ASD and SUD, such as common elements of circuitry supply and the pathophysiology of both autism and addictive behaviors. Research addressing underlying dopamine and oxytocin dysregulation in individuals with either diagnosis indicate that individuals with autism or addiction disorders may respond to rewards differently than the general population.[22]

Perceived Protective and Risk Factors

Particular characteristics of patients with autism might be seen as protective factors for developing an SUD. Social and communication challenges, sensory sensitivities, a desire for structure and rule following are generally viewed as barriers against developing an SUD. The sensory issues of autism might lead to assumptions that there is a low risk for consuming alcohol or illicit drugs because sensory sensitivities might discourage intake. For example, someone with ASD might not be able to abide the taste of alcohol or its aftereffects. "I'm alcohol intolerant - all the types I've tried have a horrible taste/after-taste and the stuff makes me feel like crap later."[23] Sensory issues might prevent individuals with ASD from managing the feel of drug delivery nasally, intravenously, or via smoke inhalation, "I find the consumption methods disgusting ex: smoking, snorting, injecting."[24] It may also be assumed that individuals with autism do not have the social wherewithal to locate and purchase illicit substances or the communication skills to navigate the nuanced and discreet interactions necessary to purchase illegal drugs or alcohol when underage.

These assumed protective factors of ASD for preventing a SUD may be risk factors for developing an SUD. Individuals with autism often report that drugs or alcohol dampen sensory sensitivities. One vlogger reports: "… dealing with a lot of the sensory integration problems people with Asperger's sometimes have—noises being too loud, lights being too bright, too much commotion going on at once, not liking how your shirt feels on your skin … a lot of people with autism and Asperger's might use a substance to block all that shit out and that's what I did."[25] Some researchers misinterpreted individuals with ASD's social challenges, assuming these challenges indicated a lack of interest in social interaction rather than an unwanted barrier to connecting with others.[5] Most people with autism desire relationships and, like the general population, may use drugs or alcohol to help facilitate social interactions. As 1 study participant noted: ""I always used to drink before going out to social occasions, because having Aspergers you're not always comfortable in social situations."[5] This observation is also true for communication challenges, because people with autism report that substances can help facilitate social exchanges: "When I'm drunk … I'm just so much more relaxed, more sociable. I can have weird conversations with people. I walk up to people and introduce myself. People think that I'm just a normal person."[26]

CONSTRUCTED NARRATIVES
Constructed Narrative and Its Impact on Health Care

A narrative is a way of giving meaning to experience by reconciling inner beliefs with outer observations. An active blending of personal and cultural resources is at the root of narrative. Jerome Bruner[27] offers that narrative is a means of organizing experience and constructing reality. He goes on to explain, "Narratives, then, are a version of reality whose acceptability is governed by convention and 'narrative necessity' rather than by empirical verification and logical requiredness…"[27(p4)] With that definition of narrative in mind, for the purpose of this article, constructed narratives have an additional layer of culturally constructed meaning. Essentially, constructed narratives form once a culture or society upholds and maintains a particular version of a narrative's reality until it takes hold.[28(p106)] A constructed narrative is often propagated in order to bolster political aims. One example might be after 9/11, when the acts of a few radicalized Muslims became part of a constructed narrative that had an impact on all Muslims.

The Constructed Narrative of Autism Spectrum Disorder

It is common for individuals with disabilities, particularly developmental disabilities, to be infantilized.[29] These narratives may evolve benignly but, left unchecked, they can inadvertently propagate stereotypes, stigma, and prejudice that can be exceedingly harmful. Adolescents or adults with autism are often portrayed as innocent or naive. People with ASD are regularly described as childlike and guileless, unable to lie and easily taken advantage of.[30] Although this narrative may be accurate in some cases, it can be overused and misleading. For example, the much-lauded television series, *Atypical*, about a high school student with ASD and his neurotypical desires, propagates the cultural narrative of an individual with autism as an innocent used as a foil to neurotypicals in order to offer the audience a bit of humor and just enough transgression for some family-friendly shock. The program's official trailer ends with the adolescent with autism sitting in the passenger seat of his mother's car. As she drives he states: "At some point, I really, really hope I get to see boobs."[31] The mother's straight face shifts to an expression that is a mix of surprise and dismay. The viewers are all in on the joke. The person with autism's direct and unfiltered verbal expression of sexual desire is akin to the desire of an 8-year-old: so sweet, so guileless, and, ultimately, desexualized. This narrative has some basis: individuals with autism may lack nuanced social or communication skills that could filter or phrase their desires subtly. However, what if this high school student expressed the same desire in adult slang? If he had, how would it have been received? If the series hero had said "I really, really hope I get to see tits" while sitting next to his mother, the narrative would become a little more dangerous, a bit frightening, and perverted. Although equally accurate, it does not fit in with society's construction of an individual with disabilities, particularly developmental disabilities, safely expressing sexual desire in a childlike manner, essentially desexualized.[32]

The Constructed Narrative of Substance Use Disorder

What about the narrative associated with someone who has an SUD? Innocent and guileless would probably not be the adjectives that come to mind. The narrative linked to those with SUD is usually one of dangerousness, dishonesty, and corruption.[33] No doubt the criminalizing of this medical condition has significantly influenced its narrative. The cultural construction of the person in active addiction is someone who has no scruples, no morals, and no compassion, rather than someone struggling to survive.

Like *Atypical*, the television series *Nurse Jackie* about a dedicated nurse who struggles with an opioid addiction is said to offer a grounded, compassionate, and understanding portrayal of someone with a diagnosis of SUD, essentially debunking the cultural construction of the addict. The official trailer for *Nurse Jackie* ends with, "Walking the line between saint and sinner, Edie Falco is Nurse Jackie…"[34] Instead of lessening stigma, the narrative of addiction could not be clearer: Nurse = saint, nurse with SUD = sinner. Again, this narrative would be seen differently if the tag line had been: "Walking the line between helper and sufferer" or "provider and patient" or "saint and substance user, Edie Falco is…"

The 2 narratives surrounding autism and addiction are not expected to converge, and they do not. That is to say that the dearth of concern, research, and action in relation to the dual diagnosis of ASD and SUD is most likely caused by each narrative's disconnection from the other. A 2016 literature review of the few publications addressing co-occurring ASD and SUD concluded that screening for substance use is standard practice for most mental health diagnoses but far less routine for those with an autism diagnosis.[3]

An Example of an Accepted Intersection of Constructed Narratives

Why is SUD screening a standard practice for most mental health diagnoses but not autism? Individuals with autism share a variety of symptoms and challenges with those diagnosed with schizophrenia. However, there is significantly more research addressing a schizophrenia/SUD dual diagnoses than one of ASD/SUD, even though an autism diagnosis is more prevalent than a diagnosis of schizophrenia.[35,36] Although other factors could be at play, such as high-functioning autism's late arrival in the early 1990s to the disorder's diagnostic criteria, from a constructed narrative perspective, the discrepancy is most likely caused by the narrative associated with schizophrenia being more in line with that for SUD. This connection is particularly provocative because patients diagnosed with schizophrenia have eccentricities and social challenges similar to individuals with an autism diagnosis, but the constructed narratives associated with both diagnoses are considerably different.[37] For example, even though individuals with autism and schizophrenia diagnoses may be equally represented in the criminal justice system, the diagnosis of schizophrenia is more likely than autism to evoke a cultural narrative of danger and uncontrolled violence.[38,39] Of course, this narrative is inaccurate: clinical research clearly shows that people with schizophrenia are significantly more likely to be the victim of violence than the perpetrator, but the constructed narrative allows a connection between schizophrenia and SUD to be accepted.[40] The narratives of both schizophrenia and SUD align and so the medical community has been able to accept and endorse the connection, giving it significantly more attention than a dual diagnosis of ASD and SUD. The unintended consequence of the endorsement of schizophrenia's and SUD's common narrative tropes could be a robust body of research addressing the connection between the two.[41] However, the lack of convergence of the ASD and SUD narratives has led to a paucity of research, even though addiction to substances is just as serious a problem for the ASD community.

ASSESSMENT AND TREATMENT OPTIONS

There is significant evidence that SUD should be a concern within the autism community and the medical community, but there is minimal attention being paid to this dual diagnosis. There are a very few studies addressing treatment, and those that do have very small sample sizes. In addition, for the most part, the treatment is not particularly innovative. Most of the literature recommends a team approach and collaboration among providers from both the autism and recovery communities.

Screenings and Assessments

The Diagnostic and Statistical Manual of Mental Disorders, Fifth Revision, cross-cutting symptom measure is a 23-question self-rated and informant-rated health assessment with 2 questions dedicated to substance use/misuse.[42] If an individual's scores on either of those questions raises concern, the ASSIST screening tool is recommended.[42] Although the alcohol, smoking and substance involvement screening test (ASSIST) is thorough and easy to understand, many of the questions are predicated on someone who has had successes that are now compromised because of substance use. An adult with autism may not have the same baseline as someone who is neurotypical, and so the answers to questions such as "During the past 3 months, how often have you failed to do what was normally expected of you because of your use of (FIRST DRUG, SECOND DRUG, AND SO FORTH)?" or "Has a friend or anyone else ever expressed concern about your use of (FIRST DRUG, SECOND DRUG, AND SO FORTH)?" may not reveal as much information as intended.[43]

Some providers recommend the car, relax, alone, forget, friends, trouble.(CRAFFT), a screening tool used for teenage substance use, with its simple wording and yes-or-no answer format, the CRAFFT could be a good fit for individuals with ASD who have concrete thinking and would benefit from simple yes-or-no questions.[44] The CRAFFT's queries "Do you ever use alcohol or drugs to relax, feel better about yourself, or fit in?" or "Do you ever use alcohol or drugs while you are by yourself, or alone?" may also be a good fit for patients with social and intellectual challenges.

Whatever screening tools providers choose, they need to read them first to ensure that the language is clear and direct. For example, questions such as, "Have people annoyed you by criticizing your drinking?" or "Have you ever had a drink first thing in the morning to steady your nerves or to get rid of a hangover (eye-opener)?" from the often-used CAGE (cut- annoyed-guilty- eye) screening tool might need to be reworded to something like, "Do people complain about your drinking? Does their complaining annoy you?" or "Do you sometimes wake up nervous or shaking? Does drinking make it stop?"[45]

Individuals with ASD may be more comfortable with online screening tools. Again, providers need to be aware that the questions can be unclear. Some online tools have questions such as, "Do you use more than 1 drug at a time?" which might be confusing if medications are being prescribed. The tobacco, alcohol, prescription medication, and other substance use (TAPS) is an online tool that is simple and straightforward, is meant to be done with a health care professional present, and can be completed by either the patient or the clinician.[46] Once the screening is complete, the outcomes include clear and detailed recommendations for how a clinician might move forward with the patient, including links to recommended interventions. The National Institute on Drug Abuse Screening and Assessment Tool Chart has links to a variety of evidence-based screening and assessment tools and resource materials for both adults and adolescents (although not specifically for those with ASD) that are easy to access and explore.[47]

Treatment Options

The 1 evidence-based treatment that overlaps for both diagnoses is cognitive behavior therapy (CBT), and 1 study cites that patients benefitted when SUD treatment providers were educated about ASD and then trained in CBT adapted to ASD.[48] The study's CBT protocols were based on adaptations by Wood and colleagues[49] that maintain traditional CBT goals such as exposing and challenging irrational beliefs while adding behavioral support and other treatment elements tailored specifically for ASD. Although Wood and colleagues[49] promote using a manual, Helverschou and colleagues'[48] explorative study of CBT for co-occurring ASD and SUD found the needs of the participants too complex to simply follow a manualized CBT format, and instead providers adapted their treatment according to each individual's particular strengths and challenges. Despite the call for flexibility and creativity, the study recommends treatment be structured, direct, and concrete. Supplemental written instructions are also recommended. In order to add predictability and reduce anxiety, providers are encouraged to regularly clarify duration of treatment and keep to a set schedule. Another recommended component of treatment is psychoeducation for both the providers and the patients regarding the characteristics of ASD and their impact. Study results emphasize that supervision for the SUD providers is critical because they may think they are incompetent because of their lack of familiarity with ASD. The biggest takeaway of this study seems to be less about CBT as a stand-alone treatment protocol and more about the necessity of collaboration among SUD, ASD, and area services providers, emphasizing significant and ongoing community support (eg, housing and employment opportunities) during and after treatment to achieve and sustain positive outcomes. Wraparound services to improve individuals' quality of life and maintain recovery have been a consistent long-term rallying cry of SUD providers for their clients with or without ASD.[50]

A more novel approach to treatment appeared in a published case study that found that the usual mandated treatments for SUD, such as group therapies and fellowships, did not work for the study's participant and so the investigators tapped into the subject's desire for routine, using a tracking log to monitor and reduce use.[51] In their article "Treatment of Addiction in Adults," Lalanne and colleagues[52] advocate for various treatment modalities such as cognitive remediation therapy (CRT), an intervention that targets executive dysfunction that can accompany both excessive alcohol use and ASDs. Although there are no evidence-based studies endorsing CRT for a dual diagnosis, Lalanne and colleagues[52] found that their patients benefitted from enhancing executive function before enrolling them in traditional psychosocial therapies such as CBT to treat SUD. Another recommended approach is motivational interviewing (MI), which is not a therapy but a means of steering individuals to consider treatment by tapping into their own desire for change.[53] MI is a technique that acknowledges ambivalence in order to encourage change. The goal of MI is to resolve ambivalence toward giving up a drug of addiction by tapping into the client's desires and values. Rather than confrontation or argument, the clinician forms an alliance with the client by using empathy, understanding, and support but also direction and guidance. The patient and therapist work together collaboratively to move toward change.[53] Although MI is being explored as a technique that might be effective for patients with ASD, there seem to be no evidence-based studies endorsing its efficacy. Lalanne and colleagues[52] recommend clinicians be wary of abstract goals and motivations. Providers might need to assist a patient with verbalizing ambivalence and may need to use diagrams or other visual aids to illustrate the discrepancies between their current behaviors and their goals.

The director of transition services for University of North Carolina treatment and education of autistic and communication related handicapped children (TEACCH) autism program uses MI by folding it into TEACCH's Transition to Employment and Postsecondary Education Program (T-STEP), which is used to achieve a variety of goals.[54] SUD treatment is reframed by using T-STEP's goal-setting techniques, such as formulating a "dream goal," which may or may not be related to recovery, and distilling it into short-term objectives that include harm reduction or abstinence-based action steps. This approach treats the client's addiction as a barrier to a desired outcome rather than alcohol or drug cessation as the desired outcome. For example, if a client has a dream goal to live independently, short-term objectives could address the importance of financial autonomy via maintaining employment and saving money, both of which could be compromised by substance use. The clinician then uses MI to help the client gain understanding of how substance use might be an obstacle to achieving the long-term goal. So, if clients share that they drink until they pass out, empathetically ask the clients some questions: was the client able to make it to work on time the next day? Does the drinking affect work performance? If the client reports they make excuses for tardiness or poor job performance, the clinician can ask whether that feels honest. If not, how does being dishonest make the client feel? Does it make the client feel isolated or lonely? Using MI as a means of self-actualization can motivate individuals with SUD to consider change, and then the therapist and client can collaborate to create achievable actions steps such as cutting back on substance use for 3 weeks or trying at least 1 Alcoholics Anonymous (AA)/Narcotics Anonymous (NA) meeting a week (with or without family or support).

One role ASD professionals or their clients should expect when seeking treatment is that of interpreter to ensure that health care professionals unfamiliar with ASD are aware of the characteristics of autism and adapt protocols accordingly. If detox, inpatient, or intensive outpatient treatment (such as a partial hospitalization program) is considered, it is critical that the facility's staff understand ASD and the importance of consistency when treating someone with autism. Even though facilities should have structured schedules throughout the day, there still can be a lot of unknowns that might make it difficult for someone with ASD to adapt. For instance, in an inpatient detox facility, a doctor may prescribe a taper to treat alcohol, benzodiazepine, or opioid withdrawal without explaining how the taper works. For someone with autism, transparency could reduce anxiety because the treatment may change daily because of medications being introduced and then tapered back. Sometimes a patient's prescribed medications may be contraindicated while detoxing from the substance of addiction. For example, if the individual has had seizures in the past while detoxing from alcohol or benzodiazepines and is taking the antidepressant bupropion (Wellbutrin), the medication may be discontinued while the patient is in detox because seizures can be a side effect of bupropion.[55] These sorts of changes need to be explained in a clear and understandable manner. In inpatient treatment facilities, clinicians often meet with patients when time is available, and those meetings could vary from day to day. It may be important to educate SUD providers that clients with ASD might benefit from adding structure, such as offering a daily meeting time or a warning if a meeting time might change. In order to facilitate consistency and reduce anxiety, clinicians may want to work with the clients to create a protocol and print an agenda for their sessions that they can adhere to each time they meet. Facilities may have rounds or team meetings every other day or once a week, and, again, explaining this component to the patient in advance could reduce anxiety and allow the patient to prepare and process. It might also be helpful to educate SUD clinicians on how to coach their patients with ASD for participation in groups, because SUD treatment often adheres to group treatment protocols. It is common for those who are uncomfortable attending groups to be labeled noncompliant.[56] Individuals who attend substance abuse intensive outpatient treatment (SAIOP) may need the group process explained on when/how to share and how much to share (role playing could help). Given developmental disability, mental health, and substance use services are often siloed, educating SUD providers about social, communication, and sensory challenges might allow more considered treatment and follow-up care for individuals with autism.

Family interventions are traditionally stressed more for autism interventions than addiction treatment. In their article on treatment of addictions for adults with ASD, Lalanne and colleagues[52] advocate family interventions. Most SUD treatment facilities tend to separate the individual from the family while the patient is in treatment and might, toward the end of treatment, cautiously reintroduce family back into the process. The National Institute for Drug Abuse endorses several family-based treatment modalities for SUD. Including family while treating both diagnoses makes sense because treatment can reduce stress for the family, which ultimately benefits the patient. Families may also benefit from clinical counsel as they navigate the fine line between support and enabling, particularly for families used to autism early-intervention treatments. Family members may also need guidance on how to support recovery; it is common for family to inadvertently push the person with an SUD back to using.[57]

Although for-profit residential addiction treatment providers tout tailored treatments for patients with co-occurring disorders including autism, there seems to be no evidence of their effectiveness.

Peer Support Groups and Fellowships

There are no studies regarding the efficacy of fellowships such as AA, NA, SMART (Self-Management and Recovery Training), or Refuge Recovery for individuals with autism. In addition, the evidence for some peer group outcomes, such as AA, is mixed for the general population.[58] Anecdotally, individuals with ASD post that these fellowships' rules bring a welcomed structure and the meetings offer a much-needed social network, or they complain about AA's or NA's rigidity, a religious/cultish/judgmental feel, and the ritual of the meetings, not understanding the process and the unspoken rules.[59] SMART recovery, a fellowship rooted in CBT, might be a good fit for someone with co-occurring ASD and SUD but it is not as ubiquitous as AA and NA. It is important to assess and reassess whether a group setting is amenable for someone with ASD. Individuals in AA joke about the 13th step, alluding to predatory behaviors of more established members toward newcomers (most often men toward women) that could be dangerous for someone that may have challenges reading social cues. Often the criminal justice system mandates individuals facing charges related to their substance use to attend group treatment, and modalities such as AA or SAIOP may not be the right fit for somebody with an autism diagnosis.

Psychopharmacologic Treatment Options

The Internet provides an array of illicit substances as treatment of ASD and SUD, with MDMA (3,4-methylenedioxymethamphetamine) and cannabis being the most common (in some locales, cannabis is not illicit anymore). Because this article is addressing substance misuse that might lead to SUD, it would be hard to justify their inclusion as possible treatment options.

Medication-assisted treatment such as methadone or buprenorphine (Subutex or Suboxone) is a highly effective treatment of opioid use disorders. The latter has had extremely positive outcomes because, unlike methadone, it can be prescribed and so does not tether individuals to their treatment.[60] There is no evidence as to any difference in effectiveness for patients with autism because there has been no research.

Acamprosate can reduce the effects of alcohol on the brain, limiting rewards and reducing cravings. Naltrexone and the long-acting monthly shot, Vivitrol, is an opioid blocker that can offer improved outcomes for both opioid use disorder as well as alcohol use disorder. There are several studies of Naltrexone as a treatment of autism (in children) with modest results.[61]

Psychopharmacologic treatments such as antidepressants or non–habit-forming antianxiety medications should be considered for underlying mental health conditions if they are contributing to substance use. It is not recommended that benzodiazepines be prescribed for someone with an SUD as they can be habit forming. If benzodiazepines are prescribed, the course should only be for a short period of time, such as a week or 2, not long term.

Although several treatment options are possible for patients with co-occurring ASD and SUD, most are not evidence based and those that have been studied, such as Helverschou and colleagues'[48] recent exploratory study of CBT or Rengit and colleagues'[51] study of the use of a tracking log, have small sample sizes and no control groups. Despite the evidence that treatment is needed, there is still no evidence-based treatment of individuals with a dual diagnosis.

SUMMARY

According to recent research, individuals with an autism diagnosis are twice as likely to develop an SUD than the general population. However, despite this research and a handful of published studies that bolster the connection between these 2 diagnoses, there does not seem to be much alarm within the autism community or the medical community at large. At present, there are a few evidence-informed treatment studies, but small sample sizes and uneven outcomes offer limited and modest options.

One means of increasing awareness is to deconstruct narratives propagated by the medical community and, more broadly, society. Respecting individuals with an autism spectrum and/or SUD and not stereotyping them by accepting constructed narratives in which the person is either innocent or dangerous, guileless or nefarious, childlike or duplicitous could help to change outcomes. Ultimately, those with both diagnoses deserve support and a decent quality of life. Deconstruction of constructed narratives is critical to overcoming biases, raising awareness, expanding preventive initiatives, increasing screenings and assessments, offering support and resources, and encouraging innovative research into the most effective treatment strategies. Both ASD and SUD have a history of inaccurate constructed narratives such as the so-called refrigerator mother as the root cause of a child's autism or the so-called crack baby as the inevitable offspring of someone struggling with cocaine use disorder. Thankfully, those descriptors have faded, but other harmful culturally constructed narratives remain. It is the duty of clinicians to continually step back, assess, and reassess and it is their responsibility to propagate narratives that are nuanced and respectful.

DISCLOSURE

The author receives (minimal) royalties from Jessica Kingsley Publishers.

REFERENCES

1. Butwicka A, Butwicka A, Långström N, et al. Increased risk for substance use-related problems in autism spectrum disorders: a population-based cohort study. J Autism Dev Disord 2017;47:80–9.

2. Santosh PJ, Mijovic A. Does pervasive developmental disorder protect children and adolescents against drug and alcohol use? Eur child Adolesc Psychiatry 2006;15(4):183–8.

3. Arnevik EA, Helverschou SB. Autism spectrum disorder and co-occurring substance use disorder - a systematic review. Subst Abuse 2016;2016:69–75.

4. Roux AM, Shattuck PT, Rast JE, et al. National autism indicators report: transition into young adulthood. In: Drexel AJ, editor. Life course outcomes research program. Philadelphia: Autism Institute, Drexel University; 2015. p. 61–63, 66.

5. Clarke T, Tickle A, Gillott A. Substance use disorder in Asperger syndrome: an investigation into the development and maintenance of substance use disorder by individuals with a diagnosis of Asperger syndrome. Int J Drug Policy 2016; 27:154–63.

6. Radliff KM, Wheaton JE, Robinson K, et al. Illuminating the relationship between bullying and substance use among middle and high school youth. Addict Behav 2012;37:569–72.

7. Center for Disease Control and Prevention. Violence prevention: preventing adverse childhood experiences. 2019. Available at: https://www.cdc.gov/violenceprevention/childabuseandneglect/aces/fastfact.html?CDC_AA_refVal=https%3A%2F%2Fwww.cdc.gov%2Fviolenceprevention%2Fchildabuseandneglect%2Facestudy%2Faboutace.html. Accessed January 7, 2020.

8. Simonoff E, Pickles A, Charman T, et al. Psychiatric disorders in children with autism spectrum disorders: prevalence, comorbidity, and associated factors in a population-derived sample. J Am Acad Child Adolesc Psychiatry 2008;47:921–9.

9. Szalavitz M. Unbroken brain: a revolutionary new way of understanding addiction. New York: St. Martin's Press; 2017.

10. Obsessions, repetitive behaviour and routines. National autistic society website; 2016. Available at: https://www.autism.org.uk/about/behaviour/obsessions-repetitive-routines.aspx. Accessed November 23, 2019.

11. Sughondhabirom A, Jain D, Gueorguieva R, et al. A paradigm to investigate the self-regulation of cocaine administration in humans. Behav Pharmacol 2005;180: 436–46.

12. Tinsley M, Hendrickx S. Asperger syndrome and alcohol: drinking to cope? London: Jessica Kingsley Publishers; 2008.

13. Sober Recovery Forums. Aspergers syndrome. Available at: http://www.soberrecovery.com/forums/mental-health/143188-aspergers-syndrome.html. Accessed April 29, 2016.

14. Reddit.com. I'm an autistic poly substance drug addict and drugs really have been the only good thing in my life. Available at: https://www.reddit.com/r/Drugs/comments/dh55sn/im_an_autistic_poly_substance_drug_addict_and/. Accessed November 23, 2019.

15. Rosie's quest Re: BOGO: self medicating and aspergers. 2013. Available at: https://www.youtube.com/user/RosieTeaflower. Accessed April 16. 2017.

16. Reddit.com. I use drugs as a coping mechanism for my aspergers. Available at: https://www.reddit.com/r/aspergers/comments/2emao6/i_use_drugs_as_a_coping_mechanism_for_my_aspergers/. Accessed December 3, 2019.

17. National Institute on Drug Abuse. Principles of adolescent substance use disorder treatment: a research-based guide. 2014. Available at: https://www.drugabuse.gov/publications/principles-adolescent-substance-use-disorder-treatment-research-based-guide/frequently-asked-questions/why-do-adolescents-take-drugs. Accessed March 13, 2017.

18. Center for Disease control and prevention. Prevent violence: prevent bullying. 2019. Available at: https://www.cdc.gov/violenceprevention/youthviolence/bullyingresearch/fastfact.html?CDC_AA_refVal=https%3A%

2F%2Fwww.cdc.gov%2Fviolenceprevention%2Fyouthviolence& percnt;2Fbullyingresearch%2Findex.html. Accessed January 7, 2020.

19. Are you autistic? Channel 4 documentary. 2018. Available at: https://www. youtube.com/watch?v=RCgPN6uFJME. Accessed June 24, 2019.

20. Autism and addiction: a problem with deep roots. Thinking person's guide to autism. Autism news and resources: from autistic people, professionals, and parents. 2018. Available at: http://www.thinkingautismguide.com/2018/07/autism-and-addiction-problem-with-deep.html. Accessed October 12, 2019.

21. Rothwell PE. Autism spectrum disorders and drug addiction: common pathways, common molecules, distinct disorders? Front Neurosci 2016;10:20.

22. Blum K, Braverman ER, Holder JM, et al. The reward deficiency syndrome: a biogenetic model for the diagnosis and treatment of impulsive, addictive and compulsive behaviors. J Psychoactive Drugs 2000;32(sup1):1–112.

23. Autism forums: an asperger's & autism community. Alcohol. 2017. Available at: https://www.autismforums.com/threads/alcohol.19726/. Accessed November 15, 2019.

24. WrongPlanet.net. Alcohol problems. 2010. Available at: https://wrongplanet.net/ forums/viewtopic.php?t=140691&p=3121851. Accessed November 15, 2019.

25. Soluna M. Asperger's and substance abuse. 2016. Available at: https://www. youtube.com/watch?v=I-Mt3VNI8RY. Accessed April 16, 2017.

26. Grant J. Aspergers Vlog-Episode 2: dealing with addiction. 2015. Available at: https://www.youtube.com/watch?v=QxBSOa-ODhE. Accessed May 8, 2018.

27. Bruner J. The narrative construction of reality. Crit Inq 1991;18:1–21.

28. Nelson HL. Damaged identities, narrative repair. Ithaca (NY): Cornell University Press; 2001.

29. Robey KL, Beckley L, Kirschner M. Implicit infantilizing attitudes about disability. J Dev Phys Disabil 2006;18:441–53.

30. Stevenson JL, Harp B, Gernsbacher MA. Infantilizing autism. Disabil Stud Q 2011;31 [pii:dsq-sds.org/article/view/1675/1596].

31. Netflix. Atypical | official trailer. 2017. Available at: https://www.youtube.com/ watch?v=ieHh4U-QYwU. Accessed November 18, 2019.

32. Murphy NA, Elias ER. Council on children with disabilities, council children disabilities, for the council on children with disabilities. sexuality of children and adolescents with developmental disabilities. Pediatrics 2006;118:398–403.

33. Room R. Stigma, social inequality and alcohol and drug use. Drug Alcohol Rev 2005;24:143–55.

34. Showtime. Nurse Jackie trailer. 2013. Available at: https://www.youtube.com/ watch?v=HB6XZu7Eav8. Accessed November 22, 2019.

35. National Institute of Mental Health. Autism spectrum disorder: prevalence of ASD. 2018. Available at: https://www.nimh.nih.gov/health/statistics/autism-spectrum-disorder-asd.shtml#part_154899. Accessed December 12, 2019.

36. National Institute of Mental Health. Schizophrenia: prevalence of schizophrenia. 2018. Available at: https://www.nimh.nih.gov/health/statistics/schizophrenia. shtml#part_154880. Accessed December 12, 2019.

37. Spek AA, Wouters SGM. Autism and schizophrenia in high functioning adults: behavioral differences and overlap. Res Autism Spectr Disord 2010;4:709–17.

38. Woodbury-Smith M, Dein K. Autism spectrum disorder (asd) and unlawful behaviour: where do we go from here? J Autism Dev Disord 2014;44:2734–41.

39. Pescosolido B, Manago B, Monahan J. Evolving public views on the likelihood of violence from people with mental illness: stigma and its consequences. Health Aff 2019;38:1735–43.
40. Angermeyer MC, Matschinger H. The stereotype of schizophrenia and its impact on discrimination against people with schizophrenia: results from a representative survey in Germany. Schizophr Bull 2004;30:1049–61.
41. Khokhar JY, Dwiel L, Henricks A, et al. The link between schizophrenia and substance use disorder: a unifying hypothesis. Schizophr Res 2017. https://doi.org/10.1016/j.schres.2017.04.016.
42. American Psychiatric Association. DSM–5 self-rated level 1 cross-cutting symptom measure, adult. 2013. Available at: https://www.psychiatry.org/psychiatrists/practice/dsm/educational-resources/assessment-measures. Accessed December 18, 2019.
43. National Institute on Drug Abuse. Resource guide: screening for drug use in general medical settings. 2012. Available at: https://www.drugabuse.gov/publications/resource-guide-screening-drug-use-in-general-medical-settings/nida-quick-screen. Accessed December 18, 2019.
44. CRAFFT.org. The CRAFFT screening interview. Available at: https://crafft.org. Accessed March 2, 2019.
45. Substance Abuse and Mental Health Administration. Stable resource toolkit: CAGE-AID – overview. Available at: https://www.integration.samhsa.gov/images/res/CAGEAID.pdf. Accessed January 8, 2020.
46. National Institute on Drug Abuse. TAPS: tobacco, alcohol, prescription medication, and other substance use tool. Available at: https://www.drugabuse.gov/taps/#/. Accessed January 8, 2020.
47. National Institute on Drug Abuse. Screening and assessment tools Chart. 2018. Available at: https://www.drugabuse.gov/nidamed-medical-health-professionals/screening-tools-resources/chart-screening-tools. Accessed January 9, 2020.
48. Helverschou SB, Brunvold AR, Arnevik EA. Treating patients with co-occurring autism spectrum disorder and substance use disorder: a clinical explorative study. Subst Abuse 2019;13. 1178221819843291.
49. Wood JJ, Ehrenreich-May J, Alessandri M, et al. Cognitive behavioral therapy for early adolescents with autism spectrum disorders and clinical anxiety: a randomized, controlled trial. Behav Ther 2015;46:7–19.
50. Faces and Voices of Recovery. 2019 public policy agenda. Available at: https://facesandvoicesofrecovery.org/about/what-we-do/public-policy/2019-public-policy-agenda/. Accessed January 8, 2020.
51. Rengit AC, McKowen JW, O'Brien J, et al. Brief report: autism spectrum disorder and substance use disorder: a review and case study. J Autism Dev Disord 2016;46:2514–9.
52. Lalanne L, Weiner L, Bertschy G. Treatment of addiction in adults with autism spectrum disorder. In: Matson JL, editor. Handbook of treatments for autism spectrum disorder. Cham (Switzerland): Springer; 2017. p. 377–95.
53. Center for Substance Abuse Treatment (U.S.). Enhancing motivation for change in substance abuse treatment. Chapter 3—motivational interviewing as a counseling style. Rockville (MD): U.S. Department. of Health and Human Services, Substance Abuse and Mental Health Services Administration, Center for Substance Abuse Treatment; 2012. Available at: https://www.ncbi.nlm.nih.gov/books/NBK64964/#__NBK64964_dtls__.
54. TEACCH Autism Program. T-STEP – TEACCH school transition to employment and postsecondary education. Available at: https://teacch.com/cllc/t-step-

teacch-school-transition-to-employment-and-postsecondary-education/.   Accessed September 23, 2019.

55. National alliance on mental illness. Bupropion (Wellbutrin). 2018. Available at: https://www.nami.org/Learn-More/Treatment/Mental-Health-Medications/bupropion-(Wellbutrin). Accessed January 9, 2020.

56. Autismhangout (dotcom). Ask Dr. Tony - addiction/depression/Jail. 2019. Available at: https://www.youtube.com/watch?v=gNYsINNE__I. Accessed July 23, 2019.

57. Center for Substance Abuse Treatment (U.S.). Substance abuse treatment and family therapy. Rockville (MD): U.S. Department of Health and Human Services, Substance Abuse and Mental Health Services Administration, Center for Substance Abuse Treatment; 2015.

58. Kownacki RJ, Shadish WR. Does alcoholics anonymous work? the results from a meta-analysis of controlled experiments. Subst Use Misuse 1999;34:1897–916.

59. Alcoholics anonymous – fitting in?. 2012. Available at: Wrongplanet.net; https://wrongplanet.net/forums/viewtopic.php?t=207993&postdays=0&postorder=asc&start=0. Accessed December 15, 2019.

60. Kakko J, Svanborg KD, Kreek MJ, et al. 1-year retention and social function after buprenorphine-assisted relapse prevention treatment for heroin dependence in Sweden: a randomised, placebo-controlled trial. Lancet 2003;361:662–8.

61. ElChaar GM, Maisch NM, Augusto LMG, et al. Efficacy and safety of naltrexone use in pediatric patients with autistic disorder. Ann Pharmacother 2006;40:1086–95.

Seizures and Epilepsy in Autism Spectrum Disorder

Frank M.C. Besag, ChB, FRCP, FRCPsych, FRCPCH[a,b,c,]*, Michael J. Vasey, BSc[a]

KEYWORDS

- Epilepsy • Seizures • Epileptic encephalopathy • Autism • Regression
- Intellectual disability • Genetics

KEY POINTS

- Epilepsy and autism frequently co-occur.
- Some epilepsy syndromes, intellectual disability, and female gender are particularly associated with the development of autism in individuals with epilepsy.
- Epilepsy and autism are likely to share common etiologies, which predispose individuals to either or both conditions.
- Genetic factors, metabolic and mitochondrial disorders, and immune dysfunction are separately implicated in the development of both conditions.
- Seizures are unlikely to cause autism in most cases.

INTRODUCTION

The relationships between epilepsy and autism have been the subject of much discussion, debate, research, and review.[1–14] Numerous studies have established beyond doubt that there is an increased rate of epilepsy in people with autism and an increased rate of autism in people with epilepsy,[9–20] although the estimates vary from study to study, depending on the diagnostic criteria used, the population examined and the methodology adopted.[4] In addition, the causal relationships between the 2 conditions are still being elucidated. Although epilepsy can cause states in which there are autistic features, for example, some types of nonconvulsive status epilepticus, the current consensus is that the co-occurrence of epilepsy and autism primarily is the result of underlying factors predisposing to both conditions. The underlying factors can include genetic conditions, metabolic disorders, infection, and other environmental influences.

This article originally appeared in *Child and Adolescent Psychiatric Clinics*, Volume 29, Issue 3, July 2020.

Funding: No funding was received in relation to the preparation of this article.

^a East London NHS Foundation Trust, 5-7 Rush Court, Bedford MK40 3JT, UK; ^b University College London, London, UK; ^c King's College London, London, UK

* Corresponding author. East London NHS Foundation Trust, 5-7 Rush Court, Bedford MK40 3JT, UK.

E-mail address: fbesag@aol.com

The purpose of this review is to provide an updated account of some of the factors contributing to the coexistence of autism spectrum disorder (ASD) and seizures.

EPIDEMIOLOGY

Although the prevalence of epilepsy has remained stable, several carefully conducted studies have shown unequivocally that the prevalence of the diagnosis of ASD has increased markedly over recent decades.[21–23] In older publications, the term, *autism*, represented the very narrow diagnostic criteria that applied to the more severe form of the condition originally described by Kanner in 1943,[24] sometimes referred to as *Kanner autism*. Recent diagnostic criteria, such as those of the *Diagnostic and Statistical Manual of Mental Disorders* (Fifth Edition) (*DSM-5*),[25] refer to "autism spectrum disorder," which has much broader diagnostic criteria. In addition, there is almost certainly much greater general awareness of autism. These 2 factors, broader diagnostic criteria and greater awareness, are very likely to be responsible for the increase in reported prevalence from a few per 10,000[26] to the latest figure from the Centers for Disease Control and Prevention of 1 in 59.[27] Why is the changing reported prevalence of autism important when considering the relationships between autism and seizures? The severe Kanner autism was much more likely to be associated with other conditions that are major risk factors for seizures, notably intellectual disability (ID). It is interesting, in this context, that the original Kanner article describing 11 children with "autistic disturbances of affective contact" included 1 child with seizures. The prevalence of epilepsy in people with severe Kanner autism is likely to be much higher than the prevalence of epilepsy in those with a diagnosis of ASD based on the *DSM-5* criteria. This is one of the factors that probably accounts for the widely reported figures for the prevalence of epilepsy in autism, namely 5% to 40%.[28] As has been pointed out by the first author of this article,[29] when quoting figures for the prevalence of epilepsy in autism, it is important to state not only the diagnostic criteria that were used but also the date of the study.

One of the most widely quoted meta-analyses is that of Amiet and colleagues.[14] This analysis highlighted the much higher prevalence of autism in those with ID (21.5%) than in those without ID (8%). Because the prevalence of epilepsy increases with increasing ID, the implication is that there is a higher prevalence of epilepsy in those with ASD who also have ID. Jokiranta and colleagues[9] confirmed that the association between epilepsy and ASD was strongest in patients with comorbid ID, especially in female patients. This association persisted, regardless of the specific ASD diagnosis (childhood autism, Asperger syndrome, or pervasive developmental disorder not otherwise specified). The US National Survey of Children's Health study for the years 2011 to 2012[30] reported an 8.6% prevalence of epilepsy in ASD; the presence of epilepsy was associated with increasing age, female gender, ID, speech problems, and lower socioeconomic status. Sundelin and colleagues[12] examined the familial risk factors relating epilepsy and ASD. Using the Swedish National Patient Register, they investigated the risk of ASD in individuals with epilepsy and their first-degree relatives; 85,201 individuals with epilepsy and their siblings (98,534 individuals) were identified, and the hazard ratios (HRs) for a future diagnosis of ASD calculated for each group compared with controls matched for age, sex, calendar period and county. During follow-up, 1381 (1.6%) individuals with epilepsy and 700 (0.2%) controls were diagnosed with ASD, yielding an HR for the diagnosis of ASD in individuals with epilepsy of 10.49 (95% CI, 9.55–11.53). Siblings and offspring of individuals with epilepsy had HRs for ASD of 1.62 (95% CI, 1.43–1.83) and 1.64 (95% CI, 1.46–1.84) respectively, compared with siblings and offspring of controls. The reverse risk, namely the risk of a diagnosis of epilepsy after a prior diagnosis of ASD, also was higher than for controls, with a reported odds ratio of 4.56 (95% CI, 4.02–5.18). The investigators concluded that ASD is more common in both siblings and offspring of individuals with epilepsy. The implication is that there are shared risk factors, which could be genetic and/or environmental. Further evidence for shared etiology emerged from a contemporary Danish study,[8] which reported an increased cross-disorder risk of epilepsy and ASD in younger siblings of children diagnosed with the alternative condition, suggesting that common genetic or environmental factors predisposed individuals to the development of either disorder. Data from the National Health Insurance Research Database of Taiwan were analyzed to determine the HRs for development of epilepsy in patients with ASD and development of ASD in patients with epilepsy, compared with age-matched and gender-matched controls without each condition.[11] Individuals with a prior diagnosis of ASD had an adjusted HR for epilepsy of 8.4 (95% CI, 5.5–12.7) compared with controls without ASD. Individuals with preexisting epilepsy had an adjusted HR of 8.4 (95% CI, 6.2–11.4) for subsequent development of ASD. A recent meta-analysis[31] determined a pooled prevalence of ASD in people with epilepsy of 6.3% from 19 studies. Particular risk factors were ID, female gender, age under 18 years, and symptomatic epilepsy.

GENETIC FACTORS

The extensive research that has been carried out on the genetic factors predisposing to autism has yielded an increasingly complex series of results. This was epitomized by the title of an article by Betancur,[32] "Etiologic Heterogeneity in Autism Spectrum Disorders: More Than 100 Genetic and Genomic Disorders and Still Counting." Included in these studies have been those that have examined genetic factors associated with individuals who have both ASD and epilepsy. Genetic defects often are associated with a wide range of expressivity; among those that are discussed in this article, many can be associated with ASD, epilepsy, and ID, in at least some individuals.

There is evidence for ASD etiologies based on complex inheritance; de novo mutations, including copy number variants; single nucleotide polymorphisms; and epigenetic variations.[33] Many of these variants are related to synapse formation, neurotransmitter function, and neuronal plasticity,[34] which is likely to explain a concurrent association with the development of neurologic disorders, including epilepsy. Advances in genetic sequencing have expanded knowledge of the genetic basis for some forms of epilepsy, in particular the epileptic encephalopathies, and have resulted in the identification of gene variants implicated in neurologic disease that also may predispose to cognitive or behavioral impairments.[35,36] Several recent reviews have attempted to catalog common genetic variants revealed in genomic and exomic studies.[2,5,33,37–40]

The concept of epileptic encephalopathy is discussed later. Srivastava and Salin[33] have comprehensively documented the known genetic convergences between epileptic encephalopathies, such as Landau-Kleffner syndrome (LKS), infantile spasms (IS), and Dravet syndrome (DS), and ASD. Mutations in GRIN2A, CDKL5, SCN1A, SLC6A1, HCN1, and SIK1, genes associated with neuronal development, ion channel regulation, and neurotransmitter function, are associated with several epilepsy syndromes, including DS, juvenile myoclonic epilepsy, IS, and Ohtahara syndrome, and the co-occurrence of ASD symptomatology with various degrees of severity.[41] True prevalence rates for ASD are difficult to determine from the original studies, however. Overall, of 62 genes with known associations with epileptic encephalopathies selected from an original survey by McTague and colleagues,[42] 32 were identified as risk factors for ASD.

Several copy number variants (CNVs) are associated with epilepsy and ASD, including 1q21 deletions, 7q11.23 deletions, 15q11.1-q13.3 duplications, 16p11.2 deletions, 7q11.23 duplications, 18q12.1 duplications, and 22q11.2 deletions, among others. A review of chromosomal abnormalities identified shared risk factors for neurodevelopmental disorders (ASD and attention-deficit/hyperactivity disorder) and comorbid epilepsy[39]; subsets of genes responsible for synaptic formation and function, namely NRX1, CNTN4, DCLK2, CNTNAP2, TRIM32, ASTN2, CTNTN5, and SYN1, and for neurotransmission, namely SYNGAP1, GABRG1, and CHRNA7, and 1 gene involved in DNA methylation and chromatin remodeling, MBD5, were highlighted. Among other shared genetic markers, variants of CLCN2, a gene associated with the formation of chlorine ion channels, and PRICKLE1, responsible for encoding the prickle homolog 1 protein, have been identified in recent exome sequencing studies of individuals with ASD.[43] Both of these genes have known associations with epilepsy. Haploinsufficiency of CHD2, responsible for chromodomain DNA helicase protein 2 synthesis, has been identified in individuals with a broad spectrum of cognitive, behavioral, and developmental deficits, including epilepsy, autistic features, and ID.[44]

SPECIFIC GENETIC SYNDROMES
Fragile X Syndrome

The fragile X syndrome is the most common inherited form of ID, which occurs as a result of CCG repeat expansions in the FMR1 gene. It usually is associated with several dysmorphic features, including a long face, large prominent ears, and a prominent jaw and forehead. Male patients are more severely affected than female patients. Estimates suggest that between 15% and 60% of patients with fragile X syndrome have comorbid ASD,[45] the wide range attributed to differences in diagnostic criteria. Seizures are a feature of between 10% and 40% of cases of fragile X.[46] FRM1 knockout mice exhibit overactivation of cortical glutamate receptor signaling[47] in parallel with abnormally decreased expression of γ-aminobutyric acid (GABA) receptors,[48] leading to dysregulation of inhibitory circuits and hyperexcitation as well as functional deficits in amygdala inhibitory synapses, with possible implications for emotional and social cognitive processes.[49]

Rett Syndrome

Rett syndrome occurs only in girls. It is clinically characterized by normal early development until the ages of 6 months to 18 months followed by a loss of language skills and purposeful hand use.[50] Characteristic hand-wringing or other hand movements replace useful hand function. It is associated primarily with mutations of the X-linked methyl-CpG binding protein 2 (MeCP2) gene. MECP2 is involved in gene regulation, in particular in a set of genes responsible for maintaining normal synaptic function. GABRB3, coding for GABA_A receptors, and DLX5, which regulates GABA production, are among the genes affected. Epilepsy and autistic features or full autism frequently develop in later stages, with up to 90% of individuals developing seizures.[51] Murine models of Rett syndrome exhibit a tendency toward cortical inhibition, which is likely responsible for cognitive and motor dysfunction, and hippocampal hyperexcitability, which is linked to seizures.[52]

Angelman Syndrome

Angelman syndrome (happy puppet syndrome) is associated with severe ID, absent speech, autistic behavior, and epilepsy.[53] It arises from a deficit in chromosome 15. The term, happy puppet syndrome, refers to the tendency to laughter, accompanied by cerebellar ataxia. Seizures and abnormal electroencephalogram (EEG), character-ized by slow spike-and-wave activity, are present in at least 80% of individuals.[54] Genetically, Angelman syndrome is associated with several abnormalities, including de-letions involving the UBE3A gene. This gene is responsible for synaptic protein synthesis and degradation; it consequently plays a role in maintaining synaptic plasticity. Loss of plasticity is associated with memory impairment and motor dysfunction in the UBE3A knockout mouse model of Angelman syndrome. Loss of inhibitory function also is asso-ciated with loss of UBE3A, which may contribute to seizure susceptibility.[53]

Although there is no suggestion that seizures are directly responsible for the autistic features seen in these disorders, the high rate of co-occurrence of epilepsy and ASD and the prominence of genetic markers associated with impaired synaptic function and excitatory-inhibitory balance provide further evidence of common etiologies.

Tuberous Sclerosis Complex

Tuberous sclerosis complex (TSC) is a disorder of cell growth regulation that results in noncancerous growths in several organs, including the brain. It arises from a genetic defect in hamartin (TSC1) or tuberin (TSC2) on chromosome 9 or chromosome 16, respectively. Characteristic facial fibromas usually develop in a distribution across both cheeks and the chin. Lesions in the kidney and lungs can cause serious prob-lems. Brain lesions can result in epilepsy, classically IS, ID, and autism. Autism may be present in up to 61% of children with TSC[55]; there is an association between ASD, the onset of seizures before the age of 1 year,[55,56] and the presence of IS.[55] Chil-dren with TSC and IS show signs of developmental delay, and higher seizure fre-quency has been shown to correlate with poorer outcomes in developmental assessments at all stages up to the age of 24 months, particularly during the first 12 months of life.[56] The presence of IS, however, does not always predict the devel-opment of ASD in TSC, and some patients develop ASD in the absence of spasms whereas patients with spasms do not necessarily develop ASD.[57] Similarly, prompt intervention to treat spasms does not always improve neurodevelopmental out-comes,[58] although a study in which children with TSC and IS were treated with the antiseizure drug vigabatrin reported an increase in mental age, suggesting a direct contribution of seizures/epileptiform abnormality to cognitive impairments, underlining the benefit of early effective treatment.[59] Other studies have suggested that antisei-zure medication may improve behavioral disturbances.[60,61] More recently, the mammalian target of rapamycin inhibitors, everolimus (Afinitor [Novartis]) and siroli-mus (rapamycin) (Rapamune [Pfizer]), have emerged as novel treatments for seizures in TSC.[62–64] In some cases, patients also have shown improvement in autistic fea-tures, behavior, and depression.[64] More generally, however, studies demonstrating improvements in social, language, cognitive, or behavioral outcomes in patients with epilepsy treated with antiseizure drugs are lacking.

A recent study by Jeste and colleagues[65] investigated the autism profile of children with TSC and found that features of social communication impairment, including ges-tures, pointing, eye contact, responsive social smile, and shared enjoyment, showed close correspondence with those seen in nonsyndromal ASD.

EPILEPTIC ENCEPHALOPATHIES AND THE ROLE OF EPILEPSY/EPILEPTIFORM ABNORMALITIES IN AUTISM

There is a stark, and in some cases potentially misleading, association between several childhood epileptic syndromes and comorbid autistic features. Berg and col-leagues[66] defined the term, *epileptic encephalopathy*, as a condition in which the epileptic activity itself contributes to severe cognitive and behavioral impairments above and beyond what might be expected from the underlying pathology alone (eg, cortical malformation). The risk of ASD or autism-like features often is substantially elevated, and some disorders additionally are associated with loss of skills that may resemble autistic regression. A systematic review and meta-analysis by Strasser and colleagues[31] determined risk of ASD by epilepsy type and reported prevalence figures of 4.7%, 19.9%, 41.9%, and 47.4% for general epilepsy, IS, focal epilepsy, and DS, respectively.

The hypothesis is that the epileptiform activity associated with these syndromes may disrupt neurologic development by altering neuronal structure or through dysregulation of neurotransmitter function.[67] There remains some controversy, however, surrounding the exact contribution that seizures/epileptiform abnormalities may make to the development and severity of autistic features in patients with epilepsy or whether a causal relationship may exist with respect to the ASD-like symptoms associated with some epileptic syndromes.

In some syndromes, for example, the LKS and nonconvulsive status epilepticus, seizures, and epileptiform discharges are related to the emergence of social cognitive and communication impairments that resemble autistic features. The development of the deficits in nonconvulsive status epilepticus is temporally associated with the abnormal electrophysiologic activity and they are not synonymous with the chronic pervasive developmental impairments that characterize ASD. Effective treatment of the seizures and epileptiform abnormalities in these cases may result in remission or resolution of the corresponding autistic features. LKS is typified clinically by a developmental trajectory characterized by normal early development of language ability followed by regression, apparently in parallel with the emergence of electrical status epilepticus of slow-wave sleep (ESES). The association between epileptiform activity and loss of communication skills in LKS, even in the absence of overt seizures, has prompted research into the possibility of a similar association in classical autism in patients without clinical seizures. A study by Baird and colleagues[21] did not find evidence of a significant difference in epileptiform EEG abnormalities between children with ASD who regressed and those who did not, although there was a trend toward a greater number in children with regression. None of the children showed evidence of ESES. Likewise, 2 recent meta-analyses by Barger and colleagues[68] found only a weak association between epilepsy or atypical epileptiform EEG and regression in children with autism, although children who regressed were more likely to have epilepsy (odds ratio 1.59; 95% CI 1.31–1.95) or an atypical epileptiform EEG (odds ratio 1.29; 95% CI, 1.09–1.52) than children who did not regress. Results from a small number of recent studies also have found that epilepsy and/or epileptiform abnormalities are related to regression. Shubrata and colleagues[69] reported that regression of developmental milestones in 25 children with pervasive developmental disorder was associated with the presence of epilepsy and an epileptiform EEG. Gadow and colleagues[70] found that reported regression in children between the ages of 18 months and 36 months was associated with epilepsy, ID, educational setting, more severe impairments in communication, and more severe schizophrenia spectrum symptoms.

Early-onset epileptic syndromes, such as DS and IS, are associated with a particularly high risk of autistic features and autism.[31] DS is a severe epileptic encephalopathy, characterized by refractory seizures, developmental delay, ID, and speech and motor impairments.[71] EEG abnormalities emerge toward the end of the first year and progress to generalized spike-waves and focal or multifocal fast spikes or polyspikes and to febrile and afebrile generalized and/or focal seizures.[71] SCN1A mutations or deletions are implicated in up to 80% of cases.[72] Most children with DS exhibit autistic features,[73] which become apparent between the ages of 1 year and 4 years in parallel with slowing or static psychomotor development.[74] Approximately 50% of patients meet diagnostic criteria for autism,[31] in a majority of cases in conjunction with profound ID.[73] The severity of cognitive and behavioral deficits may be influenced by epileptiform activity.[74–76] Studies have reported, however, that autistic features persist into adulthood, even in cases where improvements in seizures and behavioral comorbidities are seen.[77,78] A suggestion from case studies that autistic symptoms may improve when seizures are treated rigorously[79] is of interest but requires confirmation. Recent studies of cannabidiol in murine models of DS have shown improvements in seizures and autistic symptoms.[80] Cannabidiol has shown efficacy for seizures in DS in clinical trials[81–83] but its potential as a treatment of comorbid autistic symptoms remains to be established.

Between 9% and 35% of children with IS (West syndrome) develop ASD.[84] The presence of ID is an independent risk factor for autism.[19,85–87] Regression also is seen in some patients and long-term prognosis is poor. Although spasms subsequently may resolve, often other seizure types develop; for example, IS may be replaced by Lennox-Gastaut syndrome, a severe epilepsy with mixed seizure types, usually including atypical absence seizures and tonic seizures, particularly at night.[88] The emergence of autistic features in IS is notable because it occurs after the onset of spasms in the majority of cases and is apparently associated with hypsarrhythmia on the EEG.[89] More recently, however, consensus has shifted toward the opinion that etiology, rather than the presence of seizures per se, more reliably predicts the onset of ASD; individuals with symptomatic IS associated with metabolic, genetic, or structural defects are more likely to exhibit autistic symptoms than those with cryptogenic forms of the disorder.[57,58,84,90] For example, epileptiform abnormalities specifically associated with temporal lobe lesions have been identified as 1 particular factor predisposing to increased risk.[57,91,92] The presence of spasms is not in itself, however, sufficient to determine risk[57] nor does the successful treatment of seizures necessarily improve cognitive outcomes.[33,58] There is evidence that early effective intervention can mitigate developmental impairments in some cases, however,[93,94] and that prolonged untreated hypsarrhythmia is associated with poorer developmental outcomes,[95–97] underlining the necessity for early diagnosis and prompt initiation of therapy to minimize the risk of more severe long-term cognitive deficits.

In summary, despite some evidence of an apparent temporal relationship between the onset of epilepsy and the later emergence of autistic features or ASD in children with epileptic encephalopathies, which might support a contributory role for seizures in the neurodevelopmental disorder, findings are inconsistent and it does not appear that early-life seizures necessarily are predictive of ASD or the severity of ASD features. At present, the balance of evidence weighs against seizures being the cause of ASD in a majority of cases, despite some indications to the contrary. Instead, the current consensus points toward shared underlying pathologies that are likely to predispose individuals to the development of epilepsy, ASD, or both disorders.

EXCITATORY-INHIBITORY IMBALANCE

An increasing body of research supports the hypothesis that ASD is a condition characterized by abnormal neural connectivity. Functional magnetic resonance imaging and EEG studies suggest that underconnectivity, overconnectivity, or both may be a feature of the brains of individuals with ASD.[2] As previously indicated, numerous common genetic markers associated with both epilepsy and ASD relate to genes involved in synaptic formation and neurotransmitter function.[98] Specifically, dysregulation of GABA and/or glutamate signaling in ASD have been described in several recent studies.[99–102] Epilepsy is characterized primarily as a disorder of neuronal excitability,[103] with similar abnormalities in neurotransmitter function implicated in many cases. In addition to genetic factors associated with aberrant neuronal development, some of which were discussed previously, abnormalities in metabolic and immunologic function, mineral and vitamin deficiencies, and exposure to environmental toxins, including heavy metals, such as lead and mercury, also have been identified as potential pathways leading to disruption of excitatory-inhibitory neuronal mechanisms and a resultant shift toward hyperexcitation.[3] Moreover, there is evidence of separate associations for each of these factors with the development of epilepsy and autism. Particular interest has centered on research into metabolic and immunologic dysfunction and the potential role of these conditions in the development of neurologic and behavioral disorders and of autistic features. The findings from studies in these fields are discussed later.

Several recent reviews have considered the findings from genetic and epidemiologic studies, with a particular focus on the implications for excitatory-inhibitory control of various inherited and acquired pathologies associated with epilepsy and ASD.[3,53,104,105] As stated previously, there is strong evidence of GABA receptor dysfunction and/or reduced GABA signaling in some epilepsies, and similar neurodevelopmental deficits also may contribute to the hyperexcitable neuronal states seen in some patients with ASD. Takano[53] has reviewed the neurobiological characteristics of various syndromes associated with autism, including fragile X syndrome, Rett syndrome, Prader-Willi syndrome, Angelman syndrome, neurofibromatosis type 1, and TSC, which might predispose patients with these conditions to disrupted cognitive and behavioral development. Although the genetic mutations implicated in the development of these syndromes are particular to each condition and result in neurobiological dysfunctions which differ accordingly between syndromes, each appears to culminate in a disrupted pattern of neuronal connectivity in which local homeostatic equilibrium shifts in favor of either excitation or inhibition. A better understanding of the differential influence of various GABAergic interneuron subtypes in the maintenance of neuronal homeostasis and the distinct patterns of localized hyperactivity and/or hypoactivity that may result from disruption of these mechanisms might, in future, help explain the particular autistic phenotypes associated with different epilepsy syndromes and with ASD more generally.[53,105] GABAergic inhibitory interneurons are found in particularly high densities in the peripheral neuropil space surrounding pyramidal cells in the core of neocortical minicolumn assemblies[106,107] and act to buffer the core from excitatory influences originating from adjacent minicolumns.[108] Postmortem examinations have found that individuals with ASD show reduced densities in these regions,[106] particularly in minicolumns located in the prefrontal cortex.[107] Abnormal cortical excitability in patients with autism also has been revealed in studies of sensory processing, which have reported enhanced event-related potentials[109–111] and reduced cortical gamma oscillations[112] in children with ASD during sensory processing tasks. Gamma oscillations may be critical to binding and coactivation of neuronal assemblies,[3] and attenuation of these processes may underpin deficits in visuoperceptual function and contextualizing,[113–117] among other cognitive impairments.

In a recent review, Frye and colleagues[3] considered the potential mechanisms by which excitatory-inhibitory balance may be disrupted in various conditions that appear particularly associated with epilepsy and ASD. Metabolic and immune disorders are discussed later. Among other risk factors, deficiencies in magnesium, zinc, cobalamin, and folate all may result in increased cortical excitability by effecting changes in

GABAergic and/or glutamatergic neurotransmission or neuronal sensitivity. Less clear is the role of heavy metal exposure in the pathogenesis of epilepsy, although evidence of an association between lead and mercury exposure and the development of ASD has emerged from epidemiologic studies.[3] One hypothesis suggests heavy metals may reduce cortical mitochondrial function or increase levels of reactive oxygen species, with downstream effects on excitatory-inhibitory mechanisms.[3]

METABOLIC DYSFUNCTION AND MITOCHONDRIAL DISORDERS

The high prevalence of comorbid metabolic dysfunction and mitochondrial disorders in patients with epilepsy, ASD, or both conditions recently has come under scrutiny, and the hypothesis that such disorders may represent an additional etiologic pathway to the dysregulated excitatory-inhibitory balance, described previously, has been described in detail in a recent review.[118] Mitochondrial and creatine disorders[119] and metabolic disorders involving cholesterol,[120] pyrimidine and purine, vitamins including folate[121–123] and pyridoxal-5-phosphate, and amino acids[123] including phenylalanine and tryptophan, all have been described in children with ASD or epilepsy.[118] An earlier meta-analysis found that 5% of children with ASD displayed signs of mitochondrial disease and as many as 30% manifest a degree of mitochondrial dysfunction.[124] The same study reported seizures in 41% of individuals with ASD and mitochondrial disease. Other studies have found an independent association between epilepsy and mitochondrial disease, specifically in temporal lobe epilepsy,[125] especially where seizures are treatment-refractory.[126] Furthermore, mitochondrial disease is a feature of several genetic syndromes associated with epilepsy and/or ASD, including Rett syndrome[127–129] and Angelman syndrome,[130] among others. Mitochondrial dysfunction might in itself contribute to hyperexcitability by disturbing GABAergic and glutamatergic transmission, possibly as a result of oxidative stress. The role of mitochondrial disease in mediating susceptibility to seizures and ASD alternatively may be driven by induced immune dysfunction,[131] which has been independently implicated in both disorders.[132–134]

NEUROINFLAMMATION AND THE ROLE OF NEURONAL RECEPTOR ANTIBODIES
Neuroinflammation

The role of inflammatory cytokine signaling in the brain and its implications regarding the risk of epilepsy and commonly comorbid conditions, including ASD, recently has been reviewed.[135,136] Inflammatory cytokines mediate several critical brain functions, including neurotransmitter metabolism, neuroendocrine function, and synaptic plasticity. In epilepsy, abnormally high levels of brain inflammatory markers have been observed, which either might be a result of seizures or might be epileptogenic themselves, especially when exposure occurs during gestation or in early life.[136] Moreover, studies in patients with ASD have revealed neuroinflammation to be associated with GABAergic/glutamatergic imbalance, resulting in neural excitotoxicity,[101] as well as further evidence of inflammatory dysregulation, with the discovery of high levels of proinflammatory cytokines in the spinal fluid of individuals with ASD.[137] The relevance of these inflammatory markers is still being elucidated.

Neuronal Receptor Antibodies

One of the most noteworthy developments in neurology over recent years has been the recognition of the importance of neuronal receptor antibodies, including N-methyl-D-aspartate (NMDA)-receptor antibodies and voltage-gated potassium channel complex antibodies. Disorders resulting from such antibodies can present with seizures, abnormal movements, autistic features, and autonomic disturbance. In extreme cases, coma and death may result unless prompt and effective immunosuppressant treatment is implemented. Ground-breaking research in this area has been published, in particular, by Dalmau and coworkers[138–141] in the United States and Vincent and coworkers[142–146] in the United Kingdom. It is important to recognize the clinical presentation of these disorders because, in some cases, they can mimic autistic regression. For example, Creten and colleagues[147] published a case report of a 9-year-old boy who presented with acute onset of generalized seizures with no past medical or psychiatric history. Following speech and swallowing difficulties, after 10 days, he developed a severely agitated catatonic state with opisthotonic posturing, tonic posturing of limbs, insomnia, and dyskinesia. This further developed into what was described as a robotic state, with complete mutism and negativism, not responding to any form of contact. A provisional diagnosis of acute late-onset autism was made. The correct diagnosis, however, was anti-NMDA receptor antibody encephalitis. As indicated previously, the importance of recognizing such disorders is that early effective immunosuppressive treatment can result in a very good clinical response, whereas delay in diagnosis can result in serious sequelae.

SUMMARY

Although the close association between epilepsy and autism is now well established, the complexities of the relationship are still to be elucidated fully. Recent advances in genetic sequencing have further underlined the growing consensus that shared etiologies are likely to explain the frequent co-occurrence of these disorders in most cases. Aside from genetic abnormalities, recent studies have identified metabolic and mitochondrial disorders, immune dysfunction, mineral and vitamin deficiencies, and exposure to environmental toxins as possible predisposing risk factors common to both conditions. Early diagnosis of treatable conditions may be critical in determining neurodevelopmental outcome. This applies, for example, in the case of mitochondrial disorders, for many of which treatments are now available or in development. Likewise, inflammatory conditions may be treatable with anti-inflammatory therapies. The role of seizures/epileptiform abnormalities in the development and severity of ASD remains controversial. Evidence, however, that early detection and effective treatment of epileptiform abnormalities in some epileptic syndromes, for example, IS, are associated with improved developmental outcomes, emphasizes the continued need for prompt screening and accurate diagnosis. Many questions remain unanswered. In the future there should be greater attention to prompt investigation as soon as any child loses skills for no identifiable reason. The investigations should include genetic and chromosomal analyses, testing for metabolic and mitochondrial disorders, screening for neuronal antibodies, and EEG recordings, including sleep and, if necessary, overnight EEG. Recent research has shown that adverse outcomes from the coexistence of epilepsy and autism can, in at least some cases, be minimized or even avoided, suggesting that, with advancing knowledge, there might be further reduction of the clinical impact of these frequently co-occurring conditions.

DISCLOSURE

The authors have nothing to disclose.

CONFLICTS OF INTEREST

F.M.C. Besag and M.J. Vasey declare that they have no conflicts of interest.

REFERENCES

1. Bernard PB, Benke TA. Early life seizures: evidence for chronic deficits linked to autism and intellectual disability across species and models. Exp Neurol 2015; 263:72–8.
2. Buckley AW, Holmes GL. Epilepsy and autism. Cold Spring Harb Perspect Med 2016;6(4):a022749.
3. Frye RE, Casanova MF, Fatemi SH, et al. Neuropathological mechanisms of seizures in autism spectrum disorder. Front Neurosci 2016;10:192.
4. Jeste SS, Tuchman R. Autism spectrum disorder and epilepsy: two sides of the same coin? J Child Neurol 2015;30(14):1963–71.
5. Lee BH, Smith T, Paciorkowski AR. Autism spectrum disorder and epilepsy: disorders with a shared biology. Epilepsy Behav 2015;47:191–201.
6. Tuchman R. Autism and cognition within epilepsy: social matters: autism and cognition within epilepsy. Epilepsy Curr 2015;15(4):202–5.
7. Tuchman R. What is the relationship between autism spectrum disorders and epilepsy? Semin Pediatr Neurol 2017;24(4):292–300.
8. Christensen J, Overgaard M, Parner ET, et al. Risk of epilepsy and autism in full and half siblings - a population-based cohort study. Epilepsia 2016;57(12): 2011–8.
9. Jokiranta E, Sourander A, Suominen A, et al. Epilepsy among children and adolescents with autism spectrum disorders: a population-based study. J Autism Dev Disord 2014;44(10):2547–57.
10. Reilly C, Atkinson P, Das KB, et al. Features of autism spectrum disorder (ASD) in childhood epilepsy: a population-based study. Epilepsy Behav 2015;42: 86–92.
11. Su C-C, Chi MH, Lin S-H, et al. Bidirectional association between autism spectrum disorder and epilepsy in child and adolescent patients: a population-based cohort study. Eur Child Adolesc Psychiatry 2016;25(9):979–87.
12. Sundelin HEK, Larsson H, Lichtenstein P, et al. Autism and epilepsy. A population-based nationwide cohort study. Neurology 2016;87(2):192–7.
13. Viscidi EW, Johnson AL, Spence SJ, et al. The association between epilepsy and autism symptoms and maladaptive behaviors in children with autism spectrum disorder. Autism 2014;18(8):996–1006.
14. Amiet C, Gourfinkel-An I, Bouzamondo A, et al. Epilepsy in autism is associated with intellectual disability and gender: evidence from a meta-analysis. Biol Psychiatry 2008;64(7):577–82.
15. Volkmar FR, Nelson DS. Seizure disorders in autism. J Am Acad Child Adolesc Psychiatry 1990;29(1):127–9.
16. Rossi PG, Parmeggiani A, Bach V, et al. EEG features and epilepsy in patients with autism. Brain Dev 1995;17(3):169–74.
17. Hara H. Autism and epilepsy: a retrospective follow-up study. Brain Dev 2007; 29(8):486–90.
18. Bolton PF, Carcani-Rathwell I, Hutton J, et al. Epilepsy in autism: features and correlates. Br J Psychiatry 2011;198(4):289–94.
19. Berg AT, Plioplys S, Tuchman R. Risk and correlates of autism spectrum disorder in children with epilepsy: a community-based study. J Child Neurol 2011;26(5): 540–7.
20. Viscidi EW, Triche EW, Pescosolido MF, et al. Clinical characteristics of children with autism spectrum disorder and co-occurring epilepsy. PLoS One 2013;8(7): e67797.

21. Baird G, Simonoff E, Pickles A, et al. Prevalence of disorders of the autism spectrum in a population cohort of children in South Thames: the special needs and autism Project (SNAP). Lancet 2006;368(9531):210–5.
22. Fombonne E. Estimated prevalence of autism spectrum conditions in Cambridgeshire is over 1%. Evid Based Ment Health 2010;13(1):32.
23. Kim YS, Fombonne E, Koh Y-J, et al. A comparison of DSM-IV pervasive developmental disorder and DSM-5 autism spectrum disorder prevalence in an epidemiologic sample. J Am Acad Child Adolesc Psychiatry 2014;53(5):500–8.
24. Kanner L. Autistic disturbances of affective contact. Nervous Child 1943;2: 217–50.
25. American Psychiatric Association: Diagnostic and Statistical Manual of Mental Disorders: Diagnostic and Statistical Manual of Mental Disorders. Fifth Edition. American Psychiatric Association: Arlington, VA; 2013.
26. Lotter V. Epidemiology of autistic conditions in young children. Social Psychiatry 1966;1(3):124–35.
27. Baio J, Wiggins L, Christensen DL, et al. Prevalence of autism spectrum disorder among children aged 8 years - autism and Developmental Disabilities Monitoring Network, 11 sites, United States, 2014. MMWR Surveill Summ 2018; 67(6):1–23.
28. Canitano R. Epilepsy in autism spectrum disorders. Eur Child Adolesc Psychiatry 2007;16(1):61–6.
29. Besag FMC. Current controversies in the relationships between autism and epilepsy. Epilepsy Behav 2015;47:143–6.
30. Thomas S, Hovinga ME, Rai D, et al. Brief report: prevalence of co-occurring epilepsy and autism spectrum disorder: the U.S. National Survey of Children's Health 2011–2012. J Autism Dev Disord 2017;47(1):224–9.
31. Strasser L, Downes M, Kung J, et al. Prevalence and risk factors for autism spectrum disorder in epilepsy: a systematic review and meta-analysis. Dev Med Child Neurol 2018;60(1):19–29.
32. Betancur C. Etiological heterogeneity in autism spectrum disorders: more than 100 genetic and genomic disorders and still counting. Brain Res 2011;1380: 42–77.
33. Srivastava S, Sahin M. Autism spectrum disorder and epileptic encephalopathy: common causes, many questions. J Neurodev Disord 2017;9(1):23.
34. Bourgeron T. From the genetic architecture to synaptic plasticity in autism spectrum disorder. Nat Rev Neurosci 2015;16(9):551–63.
35. Allen AS, Berkovic SF, Cossette P, et al. De novo mutations in epileptic encephalopathies. Nature 2013;501(7466):217–21.
36. Michaud JL, Lachance M, Hamdan FF, et al. The genetic landscape of infantile spasms. Hum Mol Genet 2014;23(18):4846–58.
37. Tuchman R, Cuccaro M. Epilepsy and autism: neurodevelopmental perspective. Curr Neurol Neurosci Rep 2011;11(4):428–34.
38. Jeste SS, Geschwind DH. Disentangling the heterogeneity of autism spectrum disorder through genetic findings. Nat Rev Neurol 2014;10(2):74–81.
39. Lo-Castro A, Curatolo P. Epilepsy associated with autism and attention deficit hyperactivity disorder: is there a genetic link? Brain Dev 2014;36(3):185–93.
40. Myers CT, Mefford HC. Advancing epilepsy genetics in the genomic era. Genome Med 2015;7(1):91.
41. Hansen J, Snow C, Tuttle E, et al. De novo mutations in SIK1 cause a spectrum of developmental epilepsies. Am J Hum Genet 2015;96(4):682–90.

42. McTague A, Howell KB, Cross JH, et al. The genetic landscape of the epileptic encephalopathies of infancy and childhood. Lancet Neurol 2016;15(3):304–16.

43. Cukier HN, Dueker ND, Slifer SH, et al. Exome sequencing of extended families with autism reveals genes shared across neurodevelopmental and neuropsychiatric disorders. Mol Autism 2014;5(1):1.

44. Chénier S, Yoon G, Argiropoulos B, et al. CHD2 haploinsufficiency is associated with developmental delay, intellectual disability, epilepsy and neurobehavioural problems. J Neurodev Disord 2014;6(1):9.

45. Budimirovic DB, Kaufmann WE. What can we learn about autism from studying fragile X syndrome? Dev Neurosci 2011;33(5):379–94.

46. Berry-Kravis E, Raspa M, Loggin-Hester L, et al. Seizures in fragile X syndrome: characteristics and comorbid diagnoses. Am J Intellect Dev Disabil 2010; 115(6):461–72.

47. Dölen G, Bear MF. Role for metabotropic glutamate receptor 5 (mGluR5) in the pathogenesis of fragile X syndrome. J Physiol 2008;586(6):1503–8.

48. D'Hulst C, De Geest N, Reeve SP, et al. Decreased expression of the GABA$_A$ receptor in fragile X syndrome. Brain Res 2006;1121(1):238–45.

49. Olmos-Serrano JL, Paluszkiewicz SM, Martin BS, et al. Defective GABAergic neurotransmission and pharmacological rescue of neuronal hyperexcitability in the amygdala in a mouse model of fragile X syndrome. J Neurosci 2010; 30(29):9929–38.

50. Amir RE, Van den Veyver IB, Wan M, et al. Rett syndrome is caused by mutations in X-linked MECP2, encoding methyl-CpG-binding protein 2. Nat Genet 1999;23(2):185–8.

51. Steffenburg U, Hagberg G, Hagberg B. Epilepsy in a representative series of Rett syndrome. Acta Paediatr 2001;90(1):34–9.

52. Calfa G, Li W, Rutherford JM, et al. Excitation/inhibition imbalance and impaired synaptic inhibition in hippocampal area CA3 of Mecp2 knockout mice. Hippocampus 2015;25(2):159–68.

53. Takano T. Interneuron dysfunction in syndromic autism: recent advances. Dev Neurosci 2015;37(6):467–75.

54. Williams CA, Angelman H, Clayton-Smith J, et al. Angelman syndrome: consensus for diagnostic criteria. Am J Med Genet 1995;56(2):237–8.

55. Vignoli A, La Briola F, Peron A, et al. Autism spectrum disorder in tuberous sclerosis complex: searching for risk markers. Orphanet J Rare Dis 2015;10(1):154.

56. Capal JK, Bernardino-Cuesta B, Horn PS, et al. Influence of seizures on early development in tuberous sclerosis complex. Epilepsy Behav 2017;70:245–52.

57. Bolton PF, Park RJ, Higgins JNP, et al. Neuro-epileptic determinants of autism spectrum disorders in tuberous sclerosis complex. Brain 2002;125(6):1247–55.

58. Bitton JY, Demos M, Elkouby K, et al. Does treatment have an impact on incidence and risk factors for autism spectrum disorders in children with infantile spasms? Epilepsia 2015;56(6):856–63.

59. Jambaqué I, Chiron C, Dumas C, et al. Mental and behavioural outcome of infantile epilepsy treated by vigabatrin in tuberous sclerosis patients. Epilepsy Res 2000;38(2):151–60.

60. Tuchman R. AEDs and psychotropic drugs in children with autism and epilepsy. Ment Retard Dev Disabil Res Rev 2004;10(2):135–8.

61. Di Martino A, Tuchman RF. Antiepileptic drugs: affective use in autism spectrum disorders. Pediatr Neurol 2001;25(3):199–207.

62. Canpolat M, Per H, Gumus H, et al. Rapamycin has a beneficial effect on controlling epilepsy in children with tuberous sclerosis complex: results of 7 children from a cohort of 86. Childs Nerv Syst 2014;30(2):227–40.

63. French JA, Lawson JA, Yapici Z, et al. Adjunctive everolimus therapy for treatment-resistant focal-onset seizures associated with tuberous sclerosis (EXIST-3): a phase 3, randomised, double-blind, placebo-controlled study. Lancet 2016;388(10056):2153–63.

64. Kilincaslan A, Kok B, Tekturk P, et al. Beneficial effects of everolimus on autism and attention-deficit/hyperactivity disorder symptoms in a group of patients with tuberous sclerosis complex. J Child Adolesc Psychopharmacol 2017;27(4): 383–8.

65. Jeste SS, Varcin KJ, Hellemann GS, et al. Symptom profiles of autism spectrum disorder in tuberous sclerosis complex. Neurology 2016;87(8):766–72.

66. Berg AT, Berkovic SF, Brodie MJ, et al. Revised terminology and concepts for organization of seizures and epilepsies: report of the ILAE commission on classification and terminology, 2005–2009. Epilepsia 2010;51(4):676–85.

67. Marsh ED, Brooks-Kayal AR, Porter BE. Seizures and antiepileptic drugs: does exposure alter normal brain development? Epilepsia 2006;47(12):1999–2010.

68. Barger BD, Campbell J, Simmons C. The relationship between regression in autism spectrum disorder, epilepsy, and atypical epileptiform EEGs: a meta-analytic review. Am J Intellect Dev Disabil 2017;42(1):45–60.

69. Shubrata KS, Sinha S, Seshadri SP, et al. Childhood autism spectrum disorders with and without epilepsy: clinical implications. J Child Neurol 2015;30(4): 476–82.

70. Gadow KD, Perlman G, Weber RJ. Parent-reported developmental regression in autism: epilepsy, IQ, schizophrenia spectrum symptoms, and special education. J Autism Dev Disord 2017;47(4):918–26.

71. Dravet C. Dravet syndrome history. Dev Med Child Neurol 2011;53(s2):1–6.

72. Claes LR, Deprez L, Suls A, et al. The SCN1A variant database: a novel research and diagnostic tool. Hum Mutat 2009;30(10):E904–20.

73. Li B-M, Liu X-R, Yi Y-H, et al. Autism in Dravet syndrome: prevalence, features, and relationship to the clinical characteristics of epilepsy and mental retardation. Epilepsy Behav 2011;21(3):291–5.

74. Wolff M, Cassé-Perrot C, Dravet C. Severe myoclonic epilepsy of infants (Dravet Syndrome): natural history and neuropsychological findings. Epilepsia 2006; 47(s2):45–8.

75. Dravet C, Bureau M, Oguni H, et al. Severe myoclonic epilepsy in infancy: dravet syndrome. Adv Neurol 2005;95:71–102.

76. Cassé-Perrot C, Wolff M, Dravet C. Neuropsychological aspects of severe myoclonic epilepsy in infancy. In: Jambaqué I, Lassonde M, Dulac O, editors. Neuropsychology of childhood epilepsy. Boston: Springer US; 2001. p. 131–40.

77. Berkvens JJL, Veugen I, Veendrick-Meekes MJBM, et al. Autism and behavior in adult patients with Dravet syndrome (DS). Epilepsy Behav 2015;47:11–6.

78. Catarino CB, Liu JYW, Liagkouras I, et al. Dravet syndrome as epileptic encephalopathy: evidence from long-term course and neuropathology. Brain 2011; 134(10):2982–3010.

79. Chepure AH, Somaiya MP, Subramanyam AA, et al. Epileptic encephalopathy and autism: a complex interplay. J Pediatr Neurosci 2018;13(2):273–5.

80. Kaplan JS, Stella N, Catterall WA, et al. Cannabidiol attenuates seizures and social deficits in a mouse model of Dravet syndrome. Proc Natl Acad Sci U S A 2017;114(42):11229–34.

81. Devinsky O, Cross JH, Laux L, et al. Trial of cannabidiol for drug-resistant seizures in the dravet syndrome. N Engl J Med 2017;376(21):2011–20.
82. Devinsky O, Nabbout R, Miller I, et al. Long-term cannabidiol treatment in patients with Dravet syndrome: an open-label extension trial. Epilepsia 2019; 60(2):294–302.
83. Chen JW, Borgelt LM, Blackmer AB. Cannabidiol: a new hope for patients with Dravet or Lennox-Gastaut syndromes. Ann Pharmacother 2019;53(6):603–11.
84. Saemundsen E, Ludvigsson P, Rafnsson V. Risk of autism spectrum disorders after infantile spasms: a population-based study nested in a cohort with seizures in the first year of life. Epilepsia 2008;49(11):1865–70.
85. Saemundsen E, Ludvigsson P, Hilmarsdottir I, et al. Autism spectrum disorders in children with seizures in the first year of life: a population-based study. Epilepsia 2007;48(9):1724–30.
86. Saemundsen E, Ludvigsson P, Rafnsson V. Autism spectrum disorders in children with a history of infantile spasms: a population-based study. J Child Neurol 2007;22(9):1102–7.
87. Eom S, Fisher B, Dezort C, et al. Routine developmental, autism, behavioral, and psychological screening in epilepsy care settings. Dev Med Child Neurol 2014; 56(11):1100–5.
88. Riikonen R. A long-term follow-up study of 214 children with the syndrome of infantile spasms. Neuropediatrics 1982;13(1):14–23.
89. Kayaalp L, Dervent A, Saltik S, et al. EEG abnormalities in West syndrome: correlation with the emergence of autistic features. Brain Dev 2007;29(6):336–45.
90. Askalan R, Mackay M, Brian J, et al. Prospective preliminary analysis of the development of autism and epilepsy in children with infantile spasms. J Child Neurol 2003;18(3):165–70.
91. Riikonen R, Amnell G. Psychiatric disorders in children with earlier infantile spasms. Dev Med Child Neurol 1981;23(s44):747–60.
92. Riikonen R. Long-term outcome of patients with West syndrome. Brain Dev 2001;23(7):683–7.
93. Bombardieri R, Pinci M, Moavero R, et al. Early control of seizures improves long-term outcome in children with tuberous sclerosis complex. Eur J Paediatr Neurol 2010;14(2):146–9.
94. Kivity S, Lerman P, Ariel R, et al. Long-term cognitive outcomes of a cohort of children with cryptogenic infantile spasms treated with high-dose adrenocorticotropic hormone. Epilepsia 2004;45(3):255–62.
95. Primec ZR, Stare J, Neubauer D. The risk of lower mental outcome in infantile spasms increases after three weeks of hypsarrhythmia duration. Epilepsia 2006;47(12):2202–5.
96. Goh S, Kwiatkowski DJ, Dorer DJ, et al. Infantile spasms and intellectual outcomes in children with tuberous sclerosis complex. Neurology 2005;65(2): 235–8.
97. Lombroso CT. A prospective study of infantile spasms: clinical and therapeutic correlations. Epilepsia 1983;24(2):135–58.
98. Holland KD, Hallinan BE. What causes epileptic encephalopathy in infancy? The answer may lie in our genes. Neurology 2010;75(13):1132–3.
99. Sesarini CV, Costa L, Grañana N, et al. Association between GABA(A) receptor subunit polymorphisms and autism spectrum disorder (ASD). Psychiatry Res 2015;229(1):580–2.
100. Tebartz van Elst L, Maier S, Fangmeier T, et al. Disturbed cingulate glutamate metabolism in adults with high-functioning autism spectrum disorder: evidence

in support of the excitatory/inhibitory imbalance hypothesis. Mol Psychiatry 2014;19(12):1314–25.

101. El-Ansary A, Al-Ayadhi L. GABAergic/glutamatergic imbalance relative to excessive neuroinflammation in autism spectrum disorders. J Neuroinflammation 2014;11(1):189.

102. Cellot G, Cherubini E. GABAergic signaling as therapeutic target for autism spectrum disorders. Front Pediatr 2014;2:70.

103. Barker-Haliski M, White HS. Glutamatergic mechanisms associated with seizures and epilepsy. Cold Spring Harb Perspect Med 2015;5(8):a022863.

104. Bozzi Y, Provenzano G, Casarosa S. Neurobiological bases of autism–epilepsy comorbidity: a focus on excitation/inhibition imbalance. Eur J Neurosci 2018; 47(6):534–48.

105. Jacob J. Cortical interneuron dysfunction in epilepsy associated with autism spectrum disorders. Epilepsia 2016;57(2):182–93.

106. Buxhoeveden DP, Casanova MF. The minicolumn hypothesis in neuroscience. Brain 2002;125(5):935–51.

107. Casanova MF, van Kooten I, Switala AE, et al. Abnormalities of cortical minicolumnar organization in the prefrontal lobes of autistic patients. Clin Neurosci Res 2006;6(3):127–33.

108. DeFelipe J. Chandelier cells and epilepsy. Brain 1999;122(10):1807–22.

109. Knoth IS, Vannasing P, Major P, et al. Alterations of visual and auditory evoked potentials in fragile X syndrome. Int J Dev Neurosci 2014;36:90–7.

110. Marco EJ, Hinkley LBN, Hill SS, et al. Sensory processing in autism: a review of neurophysiologic findings. Pediatr Res 2011;69(8):48–54.

111. Glaze DG. Neurophysiology of Rett syndrome. J Child Neurol 2005;20(9):740–6.

112. Uhlhaas Peter J, Singer W. Neuronal dynamics and neuropsychiatric disorders: toward a translational paradigm for dysfunctional large-scale networks. Neuron 2012;75(6):963–80.

113. Grice SJ, Spratling MW, Karmiloff-Smith A, et al. Disordered visual processing and oscillatory brain activity in autism and Williams syndrome. Neuroreport 2001;12(12):2697–700.

114. Brock JON, Brown CC, Boucher J, et al. The temporal binding deficit hypothesis of autism. Dev Psychopathol 2002;14(2):209–24.

115. Brown C, Gruber T, Boucher J, et al. Gamma abnormalities during perception of illusory figures in autism. Cortex 2005;41(3):364–76.

116. Rippon G, Brock J, Brown C, et al. Disordered connectivity in the autistic brain: challenges for the 'new psychophysiology'. Int J Psychophysiol 2007;63(2): 164–72.

117. Tommerdahl M, Tannan V, Cascio CJ, et al. Vibrotactile adaptation fails to enhance spatial localization in adults with autism. Brain Res 2007;1154:116–23.

118. Frye RE. Metabolic and mitochondrial disorders associated with epilepsy in children with autism spectrum disorder. Epilepsy Behav 2015;47:147–57.

119. Rossignol DA, Frye RE. Mitochondrial dysfunction in autism spectrum disorders: a systematic review and meta-analysis. Mol Psychiatry 2012;17(3):290–314.

120. Tierney E, Bukelis I, Thompson RE, et al. Abnormalities of cholesterol metabolism in autism spectrum disorders. Am J Med Genet B Neuropsychiatr Genet 2006;141B(6):666–8.

121. Frye RE, Sequeira JM, Quadros EV, et al. Cerebral folate receptor autoantibodies in autism spectrum disorder. Mol Psychiatry 2013;18(3):369–81.

122. Rossignol DA, Frye RE. Folate receptor alpha autoimmunity and cerebral folate deficiency in autism spectrum disorders. J Pediatr Biochem 2012;02(04): 263–71.
123. Novarino G, El-Fishawy P, Kayserili H, et al. Mutations in BCKD-kinase lead to a potentially treatable form of autism with epilepsy. Science 2012;338(6105): 394–7.
124. Frye RE, Rossignol DA. Mitochondrial dysfunction can connect the diverse medical symptoms associated with autism spectrum disorders. Pediatr Res 2011; 69(8):41–7.
125. Kudin AP, Zsurka G, Elger CE, et al. Mitochondrial involvement in temporal lobe epilepsy. Exp Neurol 2009;218(2):326–32.
126. Kunz WS. The role of mitochondria in epileptogenesis. Curr Opin Neurol 2002; 15(2):179–84.
127. Großer E, Hirt U, Janc OA, et al. Oxidative burden and mitochondrial dysfunction in a mouse model of Rett syndrome. Neurobiol Dis 2012;48(1):102–14.
128. Gibson JH, Slobedman B, Kn H, et al. Downstream targets of methyl CpG binding protein 2 and their abnormal expression in the frontal cortex of the human Rett syndrome brain. BMC Neurosci 2010;11(1):53.
129. Condie J, Goldstein J, Wainwright MS. Acquired microcephaly, regression of milestones, mitochondrial dysfunction, and episodic rigidity in a 46,XY male with a de novo MECP2 gene mutation. J Child Neurol 2010;25(5):633–6.
130. Su H, Fan W, Coskun PE, et al. Mitochondrial dysfunction in CA1 hippocampal neurons of the UBE3A deficient mouse model for Angelman syndrome. Neurosci Lett 2011;487(2):129–33.
131. Napoli E, Wong S, Hertz-Picciotto I, et al. Deficits in bioenergetics and impaired immune response in granulocytes from children with autism. Pediatrics 2014; 133(5):e1405–10.
132. Xu D, Miller S, Koh S. Immune mechanisms in epileptogenesis. Front Cell Neurosci 2013;7:195.
133. Rossignol DA, Frye RE. Evidence linking oxidative stress, mitochondrial dysfunction, and inflammation in the brain of individuals with autism. Front Physiol 2014;5:150.
134. Gesundheit B, Rosenzweig JP, Naor D, et al. Immunological and autoimmune considerations of autism spectrum disorders. J Autoimmun 2013;44:1–7.
135. Paudel YN, Shaikh MF, Shah S, et al. Role of inflammation in epilepsy and neurobehavioral comorbidities: implication for therapy. Eur J Pharmacol 2018;837: 145–55.
136. Mazarati AM, Lewis ML, Pittman QJ. Neurobehavioral comorbidities of epilepsy: role of inflammation. Epilepsia 2017;58(S3):48–56.
137. Vargas DL, Nascimbene C, Krishnan C, et al. Neuroglial activation and neuroinflammation in the brain of patients with autism. Ann Neurol 2005;57(1):67–81.
138. Dalmau J, Graus F. Antibody-mediated encephalitis. N Engl J Med 2018;378(9): 840–51.
139. Dalmau J, Geis C, Graus F. Autoantibodies to synaptic receptors and neuronal cell surface proteins in autoimmune diseases of the central nervous system. Physiol Rev 2017;97(2):839–87.
140. Spatola M, Dalmau J. Seizures and risk of epilepsy in autoimmune and other inflammatory encephalitis. Curr Opin Neurol 2017;30(3):345–53.
141. Lancaster E, Dalmau J. Neuronal autoantigens - pathogenesis, associated disorders and antibody testing. Nat Rev Neurol 2012;8(7):380–90.

142. Wright S, Vincent A. Pediatric autoimmune epileptic encephalopathies. J Child Neurol 2017;32(4):418–28.
143. Wright S, Vincent A. Progress in autoimmune epileptic encephalitis. Curr Opin Neurol 2016;29(2):151–7.
144. Varley J, Vincent A, Irani SR. Clinical and experimental studies of potentially pathogenic brain-directed autoantibodies: current knowledge and future directions. J Neurol 2015;262(4):1081–95.
145. Irani SR, Gelfand JM, Al-Diwani A, et al. Cell-surface central nervous system autoantibodies: clinical relevance and emerging paradigms. Ann Neurol 2014; 76(2):168–84.
146. Vincent A, Bien CG, Irani SR, et al. Autoantibodies associated with diseases of the CNS: new developments and future challenges. Lancet Neurol 2011;10(8): 759–72.
147. Creten C, van der Zwaan S, Blankespoor RJ, et al. Late onset autism and anti-NMDA-receptor encephalitis. Lancet 2011;378(9785):98.

Gastrointestinal Issues and Autism Spectrum Disorder

Moneek Madra, PhD[a,b], Roey Ringel[a,c], Kara Gross Margolis, MD[a,b,*]

KEYWORDS

- Gastrointestinal disorders • Autism spectrum disorders • Brain-gut axis
- Constipation • Diarrhea • Gastroesophageal reflux • Microbiome

KEY POINTS

- GI disorders are highly prevalent in ASD.
- GI disorders are highly associated with other clinical comorbidities in ASD, and must be screened for accordingly.
- Diagnosis and treatment of GI issues in ASD is challenging and often benefits from a multi-disciplinary approach.
- Large, double-blind, placebo-controlled trials are required to confirm the effectiveness of dietary and microbiome-focused therapies.

INTRODUCTION

Gastrointestinal (GI) disorders are among the most common medical conditions that are comorbid with autism spectrum disorders (ASD).[1–3] Despite their prevalence, GI disorders are often overlooked.[3] Untreated GI distress in children with ASD has been linked to many issues in this population, including sleep, behavioral, and psychiatric disorders.[4,5] It is thus essential to understand the presentations of GI problems in children with ASD. In this article we discuss the GI disorders commonly associated with ASD, how they present, and studied risk factors.

This article originally appeared in *Child and Adolescent Psychiatric Clinics*, Volume 29, Issue 3, July 2020.

Funded by: NIH. Grant number(s): NS015547.

[a] Department of Pediatrics, Morgan Stanley Children's Hospital, Columbia University Irving Medical Center, 622 West 168th Street, New York, NY 10025, USA; [b] Institute of Human Nutrition, Columbia University Irving Medical Center, 630 West 168th Street, PH1512E, New York, NY 10032, USA; [c] Columbia College, Columbia University, New York, NY, USA

* Corresponding author. Columbia University Irving Medical Center, 622 West 168th Street, New York, NY 10025.

E-mail address: kjg2133@cumc.columbia.edu

Psychiatr Clin N Am 44 (2021) 69–81
https://doi.org/10.1016/j.psc.2020.11.006
0193-953X/21/

PREVALENCE AND TYPES OF GASTROINTESTINAL DISORDERS IN CHILDREN WITH AUTISM SPECTRUM DISORDERS

GI disorders were first associated with ASD through the presentation of feeding disorders in affected children. In Kanner's[6] seminal report describing ASD, "eating problems" were identified in most children presented. Since that time, it has been found that children with ASD are up to five times more likely to develop feeding problems, such as food selectivity, food refusal, and poor oral intake, than neurodevelopmentally normal children. Food intake is also often predicated on food category and/or texture aversion.[7,8] Food selectivity in this population is often manifested as a preference for carbohydrates and processed foods.[8,9] This behavior tends to be more severe than in age-matched children and lasts past childhood.[10,11] As with other GI problems, food selectivity may be more common in ASD than in children with other causes of developmental delay.[12] GI symptoms are also more common in toddlers with ASD than children with typical development or other developmental delays,[13] implying that there may be something unique in gut development and/or function that occurs in ASD relative to not only neurotypical children but also other special needs populations.

It has been increasingly recognized that GI problems may underlie some of the feeding disorders seen in this population. In fact, the prevalence of GI symptoms in children with ASD varies from 9% to 91%.[14] The most comprehensive meta-analysis to date revealed that children with ASD were more than four-fold more likely to develop GI problems than those without ASD and, further, that constipation, diarrhea, and abdominal pain are reported most commonly.[3] Other studies have reported constipation as the primary GI comorbidity with ASD, where the odds of constipation increase with greater social impairment and less verbal ability.[15] GI disorders are also associated with increased ASD severity.[16]

Alternating constipation and diarrhea has also been reported in this population.[17] Whether this is a true alternating picture or, rather, constipation accompanied by periods of encopresis, has not been examined in prospective studies.[18] In 2010, a multi-expert panel published a consensus report on GI disorders in ASD that outlined the best practices for evaluating and treating GI disorders in children with ASD. These guidelines focused on abdominal pain, constipation, chronic diarrhea, and gastroesophageal reflux disease, which were again noted as the most common causes of GI problems in ASD.[14] The commonality of these conditions has been published in multiple studies.[3,18]

Pica, the ingestion of nonnutritive items, is also reported as a problem in children with development delays, including ASD. Pica has been associated with GI problems, such as irritable bowel syndrome and constipation, although it is not known whether the GI issues are the cause of the pica or whether the pica causes GI problems.[19] In one study, 60% of ASD patients displayed pica at some stage in their lives.[20,21] In some cases pica is associated with dangerous outcomes, including elevated blood lead levels, bezoars, obstructions, perforation, and poisoning, necessitating close monitoring of these patients.[21–24]

CLINICAL COMORBIDITIES ASSOCIATED WITH GASTROINTESTINAL DISORDERS IN AUTISM SPECTRUM DISORDERS

Of the medical comorbidities associated with ASD, seizures, sleep disorders, and psychiatric problems tend to be the conditions most commonly associated with GI dysfunction (**Fig. 1**).[5,25]

Sleep abnormalities affect 80% of children with ASD and range from reduced sleep duration to parasomnias.[26,27] Sleep disorders have been described to be associated

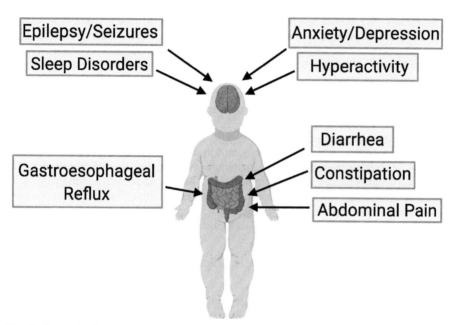

Fig. 1. The major brain and intestinal comorbidities associated with ASD.

with other psychiatric and/or other clinical comorbidities or as an autonomous issue.[28] Upper and lower GI tract problems have been associated with ASD.[29] The predominant GI conditions seen in ASD, including constipation and abdominal pain, can cause abdominal discomfort, which could be an impediment to good sleep hygiene.[14] ASD children with gastroesophageal reflux, which is also associated with GI discomfort, have higher comorbidity with sleep disorders.[30] This heightened sleep disturbance seen with GI problems in ASD children may play an important role in the quality of life for these children.

Psychiatric disorders occur in up to 70% of patients with ASD. The most common psychiatric disorder associated with ASD is anxiety,[31] although others that often present include attention-deficit/hyperactivity disorder and oppositional defiant disorder.[31] Anxiety has been highly associated with chronic GI problems in children with ASD.[32] The common manifestations of anxiety in these children include simple phobias, generalized anxiety, separation anxiety, obsessive-compulsive disorder, and social phobias. Anxiety disorders are commonly found across all levels of cognitive functioning seen in ASD.[33] These comorbidities do not differ between males and females and often persist from childhood into adolescence.[34,35]

Children with ASD and anxiety have been shown to be at greater risk for lower GI problems, which may in part be mediated through an enhanced stress response. ASD patients with GI problems have greater stress reactivity than non-ASD control subjects. Children with ASD were also shown to have greater GI symptoms correlated to higher post-stress cortisol levels.[36]

It has also been suggested that GI issues may be related to a subset of patients with autonomic nervous system dysfunction. For example, lower heart rate variability (a measure of parasympathetic activity on the heart) was associated with greater GI problems, especially in ASD patients with regression.[29] The relationship between anxiety and GI issues in ASD is an active area of investigation.[29,36]

In addition to psychiatric comorbidities, maladaptive disorders, such as irritability and social withdrawal, have also been associated with GI dysfunction in ASD.[37] Children with ASD who experience abdominal pain, gas, diarrhea, and constipation have more irritability, social withdrawal, and hyperactivity compared with those without the GI issues.[37] Argumentative, oppositional, defiant, and destructive behaviors are also more often seen in ASD children with accompanying GI problems.[5] GI distress experienced by children with ASD may thus play an important role in the behavioral problems demonstrated in this population.

Difficult and unexplained behaviors may be caused in part by the inability of some children with ASD to verbalize their discomfort in response to GI distress.[14] Consequently, GI distress may manifest in seemingly unassociated ways. For example, unexplained irritable behavior was found in 43% of ASD children with esophagitis[38] and functional constipation has been associated with rigid-compulsive behavior in children with ASD.[39] Nonverbal patients may also demonstrate GI distress as constant eating or drinking, chewing on nonedible objects, and abdominal pressure.[40]

RISK FACTORS FOR GASTROINTESTINAL DISORDERS IN AUTISM SPECTRUM DISORDERS

Although studies have identified potential genetic risk factors for ASD and GI dysfunction, most alone have been insufficient in explaining its cause. For example, a polymorphism of the MET tyrosine receptor kinase is associated with ASD and GI dysfunction in family samples, elucidating a potential genetic connection of the two pathologies.[41] Not all individuals with this genetic mutation, however, exhibit symptoms of GI dysfunction. Gene × environment interactions are likely to play a role in most etiologies.[42] Because genetic susceptibility is often elicited by environmental exposure, understanding the roles that environmental risk factors play in ASD symptomatology and/or pathogenesis is critical and an active area of investigation.[43]

Diet is an environmental factor that may affect ASD symptomatology. The most common restrictive diet used in the ASD population is one that lacks gluten and/or casein.[44] Although anecdotal reports suggest an improvement in GI and/or behavioral symptoms in individuals on gluten- and/or casein-free diets, these findings have not been confirmed in double-blind placebo-controlled trials.[45] It has also not been shown that children with ASD suffer from an increased incidence of celiac disease, wheat allergy, or milk allergy.[46] It is thus not currently recommended that children with ASD be placed on these diets indiscriminately. It is possible, however, that some children may respond positively to being on exclusionary diets, but it is not known how to identify these children or why they may benefit. There are also disadvantages to these diets; they can be highly restrictive and can thus further compound the highly selective diets children with ASD often already have.[47] A restrictive diet and picky eating can lead to nutrient deficiencies. If families are interested in trying an exclusionary diet, they should do so in close collaboration with a nutritionist.

An important way that diet may impact behavior and/or GI function is based on its ability to alter the intestinal microbiome. Diet rapidly alters gut microbiota composition and specific microbiota environments have been associated with changes in behavior, mood, cognition, and GI problems, in preclinical and clinical studies (as reviewed in Refs.[48–50]) (**Fig. 2**). Although children with ASD have been shown to have different intestinal microbiota populations than neurotypical children, the studies have been small and the results have been extremely variable.[51]

Some of the microbial differences seen in children with ASD have been associated with impaired transcription of genes involved in carbohydrate metabolism.[52] This

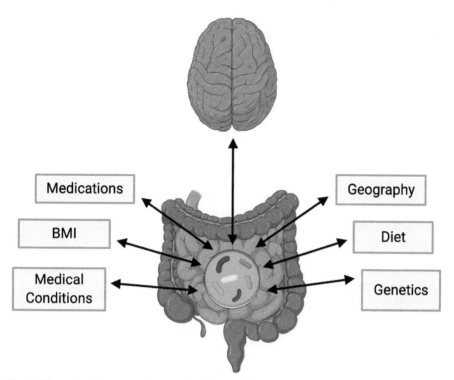

Fig. 2. The microbiome can have a significant effect on gut function and on mood and behavior. The studies that have sought to evaluate the gut microbiome in ASD have demonstrated variable results. This is likely because there are many factors that impact the microbiome that may differ, on an individual basis, in patients with ASD. These factors include diet, geography, genetics, body mass index (BMI), medications, and other medical conditions.

could thus be a reason why some kids with ASD respond poorly to gluten ingestion. There is also one report showing that children with ASD have increased immune reactivity to gluten and this immune response is enhanced when GI symptoms are present, but this study, like the aforementioned one, has not been replicated.[53] In addition to the lack of confirmatory data in this area, there are also contradictory findings; a recent study showed that dietary patterns were not associated with the GI symptoms seen in children with ASD.[54] These data are suggestive of the notion that diet is not the exclusive cause of underlying GI dysfunction in these children. Alternatively, it is also possible that subsets of children with ASD harbor abnormalities in carbohydrate digestion and/or immunity. At this point, however, it is not known whether these physiologic differences actually exist and, if they do, how physicians would be able to identify these specific patients in a reliable fashion.

Maternal factors, through prenatal exposure, have been associated with ASD occurrence. In particular, maternal obesity and gestational diabetes mellitus are two factors that have been more extensively studied and were found to be associated with a 1.5 times greater odds of ASD in exposed offspring.[55–58] In line with these clinical studies, animal research has shown that a maternal high-fat diet (HFD) is associated with gut microbiota dysbiosis, which results in changes in central neurobiology and abnormal social behaviors, linking the maternal diet and dysbiosis to neurodevelopmental disorders.[59] Studies have also shown that changing the microbiome may correct the brain and behavioral defects induced by a dysbiosis, suggesting that the intestinal microbiota may be an underlying cause of the central nervous system dysfunction in ASD and also that its manipulation could be a novel therapeutic option.[59,60] In one of these studies, administration of an HFD during gestation in mice resulted, in the pups, in a gut microbiota dysbiosis, reduced sociability, fewer oxytocin neurons in the hypothalamus, and reduced synaptic plasticity in the ventral tegmental area of offspring. A lack of *Lactobacillus reuteri* was implicated as one cause of the dysbiosis seen in this diet-induced phenotype and treatment with *L reuteri* resulted in improvements in the central nervous system and social deficits.[59] Another study showed similar results; HFD-exposed offspring expressed less vocalizations during maternal separation experiments, a measure of early life stress in the offspring, than control diet offspring. In these experiments, members of the *Firmicutes* phyla were implicated in the gut microbiome dysbiosis and behavioral correlates.[61] Recently, *L reuteri* restored social impairments in multiple ASD mouse models and novel insights into this mechanism have revealed that this process is mediated directly through the nervous system and not via changes in the gut microbiome.[60] These basic experiments have demonstrated a possible role for the gut microbiome in the generation of ASD-like phenotypes and, excitingly, possible novel treatment modalities.

Both human and animal studies have indicated an association between maternal inflammation and ASD risk.[62] The inflammation resulting from human maternal infection and/or maternal autoimmune disease has been associated with an increased prevalence of ASD in progeny.[63] Similarly, mice and/or nonhuman primates that are exposed to maternal immune activation (MIA) through maternal infection with the viral mimetic, polyinosinic:polycytidylic acid, or maternal influenza infection, have offspring that develop abnormal social behaviors,[64–66] deficits in their immune profiles, and anxiety-like phenotypes.[67] MIA has also been shown to cause increased gut permeability and gut dysbiosis.[68,69] Treatment of MIA-exposed mice with *Bacteriodes fragilis* has been shown to normalize intestinal permeability, prevent migration of neurotransmitters through the gut wall, and improve multiple hallmarks of ASD-like behaviors.[68,70] These experiments demonstrate how maternal infection may result in concomitant ASD and GI dysfunction. It is not known whether MIA-exposed pups also manifest other GI abnormalities, such as motility dysfunction or abdominal pain.

Mouse studies have shown evidence that the link between maternal inflammation and ASD development may involve placental inflammation. Placental interleukin-6, a proinflammatory cytokine, was shown to mediate the maternal infection-induced ASD risk to the developing fetus. Whereas progeny of MIA mice develop phenotypes consistent with ASD, those mice with selective deletion of interleukin-6 in placental trophoblasts had offspring that did not display these neurobiologic or behavioral abnormalities.[71] This alludes to a potential mechanism through which MIA can interfere with gestation, opening the door to future research in this area.

DIAGNOSIS AND TREATMENT OF GASTROINTESTINAL PROBLEMS IN AUTISM SPECTRUM DISORDERS

Although a reliable diagnosis of GI problems in ASD in important, they are extremely difficult to recognize because their presentations often lack the classic signs of GI distress, such as verbal complaints of abdominal pain or other signs of localization of discomfort (ie, holding of the stomach). Two of the major reasons that this occurs is because children with ASD often have limited verbal ability and, even if their verbal ability is intact, sensory perception is often abnormal, making it difficult for these individuals to localize and/or describe sources of their discomfort.[72] Consequently, children with ASD and GI pain may present with nonspecific signs or symptoms to express their discomfort, including aggression, self-injury, irritability, abnormal vocalizations (ie, frequent swallowing, moaning), motor signs (ie, grimacing, tapping), hyperactivity, changes in sleep patterns, and/or anxiety.[4,14,25,73]

The gold standard screening tool used to diagnose some of the most common pediatric GI conditions is the Rome criteria. A major problem with the Rome criteria for evaluating individuals with ASD is that its accuracy depends on the ability of the patient to speak and also to localize pain. To facilitate more accurate diagnoses in the ASD population, the Autism Treatment Network created a GI symptom inventory questionnaire to diagnose the most common GI conditions found in ASD. In contrast to the Rome criteria, GI problems were identified in this questionnaire by using observable signs for caretakers, as opposed to verbal complaints, and thus included physical behaviors associated with GI distress (ie, applying abdominal pressure). Recently, a concise version of this screening tool was created and validated. This 17-question screen, which relies on caretaker observation, was administered prospectively to caretakers and then to pediatric gastroenterologists who had evaluated the patients. Using this screen, GI problems were effectively diagnosed with a sensitivity of 86%, a specificity of 43%, and a positive predictive value of 67%. Importantly, the screen detected new diagnoses of GI problems in more than 20% of the patients.[18]

Although there are anecdotal reports of behavioral improvements following effective treatment of GI problems, prospective studies are still required.[74,75] These anecdotal reports, however, suggest that effective treatment of GI disorders is important not only for the attenuation of the GI problems, but also potential improvements in associated behavioral correlates.[74,76,77]

Treatment of GI problems in children with ASD should be addressed in the same ways as for those without ASD. Those with ASD, however, may benefit from having an interdisciplinary medical team that can diagnose and treat the different complex, and often interrelated medical conditions (noted previously) that affect this population.[14] Depending on the issues involved, a sleep specialist, psychiatrist, and/or neurologist may be most commonly useful. Nutritionists also often also need to be involved proactively in the long-term nutritional treatment strategies for these individuals.

Some of the major novel therapeutic approaches that have been evaluated in recent years in the ASD population involve manipulation of the gut microbiota. The theory that gut dysbiosis underlies some of the behavioral manifestations in ASD originated from a study in children who developed regressive ASD and diarrhea after a course of antibiotics. The study showed that short-term administration of oral vancomycin treatment resulted in improvements in behavioral correlates. Although the initial findings were promising, the behavioral improvements ceased almost immediately after the antibiotic was stopped.[78] Although not effective as a treatment, this was an important step in linking the microbiome with ASD.

Although multiple studies have shown that children with ASD have different intestinal microbiota than neurotypical children, the studies have been small with variable results.[51] The variability may be linked to the many confounding factors that can alter the microbiome (see **Fig. 2**). There are several studies, however, that demonstrate a difference in *Clostridia* levels in children with ASD, which, interestingly, is a target for vancomycin.[79–82]

Another way that the gut microbiome may be manipulated is through delivery of a fecal microbiota transplant (FMT). The one study that evaluated the efficacy of FMT in individuals with ASD showed that the patients given an FMT exhibited significantly improved GI and behavioral outcomes following fecal transfer that persisted 8 weeks post-treatment.[76] Moreover, in a recent 2-year follow-up of this same patient cohort, the GI and behavioral improvements persisted, demonstrating long-term effects of this therapy.[77] Although the results of this study are exciting, the patient sample was small (18 patients) and the trial was open-label, leaving outcomes open to the effects of placebo. An FMT study that is conducted in a larger cohort and in a double-blind, placebo-controlled manner is thus warranted.

Administration of some probiotics have resulted in improvements in ASD-like phenotypes in animal models.[68] Recently, a small, randomized pilot trial of probiotics in children with ASD and GI problems was conducted. A probiotic mixture of eight *Lactobacillus* and *Bifidobacterium* species was given for the 19-week trial period. Although parents reported a significant improvement in GI symptoms, the overall resulting quality-of-life measures were not significant.[74] In another randomized pilot study, children with ASD and GI problems were given prebiotic and probiotic treatments intermittently for 12 weeks. Although some of these patients showed improvements in GI problems and aberrant behaviors, the small sample size and lack of a true control group makes these data harder to generalize.[75] These early studies on probiotic treatment in children with ASD and GI problems thus show promise, but larger trials are necessary to better implicate the role of probiotics in ASD treatment.[14]

SUMMARY

It has become increasingly clear that GI problems are common in the ASD population and also morbidity causing. It is thus critical that clinicians understand the different presentations of GI distress in this population so efficient treatment and/or referral to a gastroenterologist can be implemented. Once GI problems are diagnosed other clinical comorbidities commonly co-occurring with GI dysfunction in ASD should also be promptly considered.

Although the treatment of GI conditions in ASD is similar in many ways to those of neurotypical individuals, additional considerations must be made. Comprehensive nutritional evaluations should be considered because of the high incidence of food aversions and the common use of exclusionary diets. Although not a currently recommended treatment, gut microbiota modulation (ie, FMT, probiotics) may be a distinct novel therapeutic option for this population in the future, as a treatment of not only GI problems but also behavioral issues.

DISCLOSURE

The authors have nothing to disclose.

REFERENCES

1. Doshi-Velez F, Ge Y, Kohane I. Comorbidity clusters in autism spectrum disorders: an electronic health record time-series analysis. Pediatrics 2014;133(1): e54–63.

2. Aldinger KA, Lane CJ, Veenstra-VanderWeele J, et al. Patterns of risk for multiple co-occurring medical conditions replicate across distinct cohorts of children with autism spectrum disorder. Autism Res 2015;8(6):771–81.

3. McElhanon BO, McCracken C, Karpen S, et al. Gastrointestinal symptoms in autism spectrum disorder: a meta-analysis. Pediatrics 2014;133(5):872–83.

4. Ferguson BJ, Dovgan K, Takahashi N, et al. The relationship among gastrointestinal symptoms, problem behaviors, and internalizing symptoms in children and adolescents with autism spectrum disorder. Front Psychiatry 2019;10:194.

5. Maenner MJ, Arneson CL, Levy SE, et al. Brief report: association between behavioral features and gastrointestinal problems among children with autism spectrum disorder. J Autism Dev Disord 2012;42(7):1520–5.

6. Kanner L. Austic disturbances of affective contact. *Acta Paedopsychiatr* 1968; 35(4):100–36.

7. Sharp WG, Berry RC, McCracken C, et al. Feeding problems and nutrient intake in children with autism spectrum disorders: a meta-analysis and comprehensive review of the literature. J Autism Dev Disord 2013;43(9):2159–73.

8. Ahearn WH, Castine T, Nault K, et al. An assessment of food acceptance in children with autism or pervasive developmental disorder-not otherwise specified. J Autism Dev Disord 2001;31(5):505–11.

9. Bandini LG, Curtin C, Phillips S, et al. Changes in food selectivity in children with autism spectrum disorder. J Autism Dev Disord 2017;47(2):439–46.

10. Cermak SA, Curtin C, Bandini LG. Food selectivity and sensory sensitivity in children with autism spectrum disorders. J Am Diet Assoc 2010;110(2):238–46.

11. Twachtman-Reilly J, Amaral SC, Zebrowski PP. Addressing feeding disorders in children on the autism spectrum in school-based settings: physiological and behavioral issues. Lang Speech Hear Serv Sch 2008;39(2):261–72.

12. Beighley JS, Matson JL, Rieske RD, et al. Food selectivity in children with and without an autism spectrum disorder: investigation of diagnosis and age. Res Dev Disabil 2013;34(10):3497–503.

13. Bresnahan M, Hornig M, Schultz AF, et al. Association of maternal report of infant and toddler gastrointestinal symptoms with autism: evidence from a prospective birth cohort. JAMA Psychiatry 2015;72(5):466–74.

14. Buie T, Campbell DB, Fuchs GJ 3rd, et al. Evaluation, diagnosis, and treatment of gastrointestinal disorders in individuals with ASDs: a consensus report. Pediatrics 2010;125(Suppl 1):S1–18.

15. Gorrindo P, Williams KC, Lee EB, et al. Gastrointestinal dysfunction in autism: parental report, clinical evaluation, and associated factors. Autism Res 2012; 5(2):101–8.

16. Wang LW, Tancredi DJ, Thomas DW. The prevalence of gastrointestinal problems in children across the United States with autism spectrum disorders from families with multiple affected members. J Dev Behav Pediatr 2011;32(5):351–60.

17. Molloy CA, Manning-Courtney P. Prevalence of chronic gastrointestinal symptoms in children with autism and autistic spectrum disorders. Autism 2003;7(2): 165–71.

18. Margolis KG, Buie TM, Turner JB, et al. Development of a brief parent-report screen for common gastrointestinal disorders in autism spectrum disorder. J Autism Dev Disord 2019;49(1):349–62.

19. Call NA, Simmons CA, Mevers JE, et al. Clinical outcomes of behavioral treatments for pica in children with developmental disabilities. J Autism Dev Disord 2015;45(7):2105–14.

20. Kinnell HG. Pica as a feature of autism. Br J Psychiatry 1985;147:80–2.

21. Cohen DJ, Johnson WT, Caparulo BK. Pica and elevated blood lead level in autistic and atypical children. Am J Dis Child 1976;130(1):47–8.

22. Serour F, Witzling M, Frenkel-Laufer D, et al. Intestinal obstruction in an autistic adolescent. Pediatr Emerg Care 2008;24(10):688–90.

23. George M, Heeney MM, Woolf AD. Encephalopathy from lead poisoning masquerading as a flu-like syndrome in an autistic child. Pediatr Emerg Care 2010;26(5):370–3.

24. Oestreich AE. Multiple magnet ingestion alert. Radiology 2004;233(2):615.

25. Kang V, Wagner GC, Ming X. Gastrointestinal dysfunction in children with autism spectrum disorders. Autism Res 2014;7(4):501–6.

26. Rossignol DA, Frye RE. Melatonin in autism spectrum disorders: a systematic review and meta-analysis. Dev Med Child Neurol 2011;53(9):783–92.

27. Mannion ALG, Healy O. An investigation of comorbid psychological disorders, sleep problems, gastrointestinal symptoms and epilepsy in children and adolescents with autism spectrum disorder. Res Autism Spectr Disord 2012;7(1):35–42.

28. Richdale AL, Schreck KA. Sleep problems in autism spectrum disorders: prevalence, nature, & possible biopsychosocial aetiologies. Sleep Med Rev 2009; 13(6):403–11.

29. Ferguson BJ, Marler S, Altstein LL, et al. Psychophysiological associations with gastrointestinal symptomatology in autism spectrum disorder. Autism Res 2017; 10(2):276–88.

30. Trickett J, Heald M, Oliver C, et al. A cross-syndrome cohort comparison of sleep disturbance in children with Smith-Magenis syndrome, Angelman syndrome, autism spectrum disorder and tuberous sclerosis complex. J Neurodev Disord 2018;10(1):9.

31. Simonoff E, Pickles A, Charman T, et al. Psychiatric disorders in children with autism spectrum disorders: prevalence, comorbidity, and associated factors in a population-derived sample. J Am Acad Child Adolesc Psychiatry 2008;47(8): 921–9.

32. Mazurek MO, Vasa RA, Kalb LG, et al. Anxiety, sensory over-responsivity, and gastrointestinal problems in children with autism spectrum disorders. J Abnorm Child Psychol 2013;41(1):165–76.

33. White SW, Oswald D, Ollendick T, et al. Anxiety in children and adolescents with autism spectrum disorders. Clin Psychol Rev 2009;29(3):216–29.

34. Hofvander B, Delorme R, Chaste P, et al. Psychiatric and psychosocial problems in adults with normal-intelligence autism spectrum disorders. BMC Psychiatry 2009;9:35.

35. Simonoff E, Jones CR, Baird G, et al. The persistence and stability of psychiatric problems in adolescents with autism spectrum disorders. J Child Psychol Psychiatry 2013;54(2):186–94.

36. Ferguson BJ, Marler S, Altstein LL, et al. Associations between cytokines, endocrine stress response, and gastrointestinal symptoms in autism spectrum disorder. Brain Behav Immun 2016;58:57–62.

37. Chaidez V, Hansen RL, Hertz-Picciotto I. Gastrointestinal problems in children with autism, developmental delays or typical development. J Autism Dev Disord 2014;44(5):1117–27.

38. Horvath K, Perman JA. Autistic disorder and gastrointestinal disease. Curr Opin Pediatr 2002;14(5):583–7.

39. Marler S, Ferguson BJ, Lee EB, et al. Association of rigid-compulsive behavior with functional constipation in autism spectrum disorder. J Autism Dev Disord 2017;47(6):1673–81.

40. Bauman ML. Medical comorbidities in autism: challenges to diagnosis and treatment. Neurotherapeutics 2010;7(3):320–7.

41. Campbell DB, Buie TM, Winter H, et al. Distinct genetic risk based on association of MET in families with co-occurring autism and gastrointestinal conditions. Pediatrics 2009;123(3):1018–24.
42. Chaste P, Leboyer M. Autism risk factors: genes, environment, and gene-environment interactions. Dialogues Clin Neurosci 2012;14(3):281–92.
43. Beversdorf DQ, Stevens HE, Jones KL. Prenatal stress, maternal immune dysregulation, and their association with autism spectrum disorders. Curr Psychiatry Rep 2018;20(9):76.
44. Perrin JM, Coury DL, Hyman SL, et al. Complementary and alternative medicine use in a large pediatric autism sample. Pediatrics 2012;130(Suppl 2):S77–82.
45. Hyman SL, Stewart PA, Foley J, et al. The gluten-free/casein-free diet: a double-blind challenge trial in children with autism. J Autism Dev Disord 2016;46(1): 205–20.
46. Buie T. The relationship of autism and gluten. Clin Ther 2013;35(5):578–83.
47. Bandini LG, Anderson SE, Curtin C, et al. Food selectivity in children with autism spectrum disorders and typically developing children. J Pediatr 2010;157(2): 259–64.
48. Murtaza N, Ó Cuív P, Morrison M. Diet and the microbiome. Gastroenterol Clin North Am 2017;46(1):49–60.
49. Vuong HE, Yano JM, Fung TC, et al. The microbiome and host behavior. Annu Rev Neurosci 2017;40:21–49.
50. Parekh PJ, Balart LA, Johnson DA. The influence of the gut microbiome on obesity, metabolic syndrome and gastrointestinal disease. Clin Transl Gastroenterol 2015;6:e91.
51. Vuong HE, Hsiao EY. Emerging roles for the gut microbiome in autism spectrum disorder. Biol Psychiatry 2017;81(5):411–23.
52. Williams BL, Hornig M, Buie T, et al. Impaired carbohydrate digestion and transport and mucosal dysbiosis in the intestines of children with autism and gastrointestinal disturbances. PLoS One 2011;6(9):e24585.
53. Lau NM, Green PH, Taylor AK, et al. Markers of celiac disease and gluten sensitivity in children with autism. PLoS One 2013;8(6):e66155.
54. Ferguson BJ, Dovgan K, Severns D, et al. Lack of associations between dietary intake and gastrointestinal symptoms in autism spectrum disorder. Front Psychiatry 2019;10:528.
55. Connolly N, Anixt J, Manning P, et al. Maternal metabolic risk factors for autism spectrum disorder: an analysis of electronic medical records and linked birth data. Autism Res 2016;9(8):829–37.
56. Li M, Fallin MD, Riley A, et al. The association of maternal obesity and diabetes with autism and other developmental disabilities. Pediatrics 2016;137(2): e20152206.
57. Xiang AH, Wang X, Martinez MP, et al. Association of maternal diabetes with autism in offspring. JAMA 2015;313(14):1425–34.
58. Modabbernia A, Velthorst E, Reichenberg A. Environmental risk factors for autism: an evidence-based review of systematic reviews and meta-analyses. Mol Autism 2017;8:13.
59. Buffington SA, Di Prisco GV, Auchtung TA, et al. Microbial reconstitution reverses maternal diet-induced social and synaptic deficits in offspring. Cell 2016;165(7): 1762–75.
60. Sgritta M, Dooling SW, Buffington SA, et al. Mechanisms underlying microbial-mediated changes in social behavior in mouse models of autism spectrum disorder. Neuron 2019;101(2):246–59.e6.

61. Bruce-Keller AJ, Fernandez-Kim SO, Townsend RL, et al. Maternal obese-type gut microbiota differentially impact cognition, anxiety and compulsive behavior in male and female offspring in mice. PLoS One 2017;12(4):e0175577.

62. Frye RE, Rossignol DA. Identification and treatment of pathophysiological comorbidities of autism spectrum disorder to achieve optimal outcomes. Clin Med Insights Pediatr 2016;10:43–56.

63. Jiang HY, Xu LL, Shao L, et al. Maternal infection during pregnancy and risk of autism spectrum disorders: a systematic review and meta-analysis. Brain Behav Immun 2016;58:165–72.

64. Shi L, Smith SE, Malkova N, et al. Activation of the maternal immune system alters cerebellar development in the offspring. Brain Behav Immun 2009;23(1):116–23.

65. Bauman MD, Iosif AM, Smith SE, et al. Activation of the maternal immune system during pregnancy alters behavioral development of rhesus monkey offspring. Biol Psychiatry 2014;75(4):332–41.

66. Shi L, Fatemi SH, Sidwell RW, et al. Maternal influenza infection causes marked behavioral and pharmacological changes in the offspring. J Neurosci 2003; 23(1):297–302.

67. Hsiao EY, McBride SW, Chow J, et al. Modeling an autism risk factor in mice leads to permanent immune dysregulation. Proc Natl Acad Sci U S A 2012;109(31): 12776–81.

68. Hsiao EY, McBride SW, Hsien S, et al. Microbiota modulate behavioral and physiological abnormalities associated with neurodevelopmental disorders. Cell 2013; 155(7):1451–63.

69. Malkova NV, Yu CZ, Hsiao EY, et al. Maternal immune activation yields offspring displaying mouse versions of the three core symptoms of autism. Brain Behav Immun 2012;26(4):607–16.

70. Mazmanian SK, Round JL, Kasper DL. A microbial symbiosis factor prevents intestinal inflammatory disease. Nature 2008;453(7195):620–5.

71. Wu WL, Hsiao EY, Yan Z, et al. The placental interleukin-6 signaling controls fetal brain development and behavior. Brain Behav Immun 2017;62:11–23.

72. Whitney DG, Shapiro DN. National prevalence of pain among children and adolescents with autism spectrum disorders. JAMA Pediatr 2019;173(12):1203–5.

73. Yang XL, Liang S, Zou MY, et al. Are gastrointestinal and sleep problems associated with behavioral symptoms of autism spectrum disorder? Psychiatry Res 2018;259:229–35.

74. Arnold LE, Luna RA, Williams K, et al. Probiotics for gastrointestinal symptoms and quality of life in autism: a placebo-controlled pilot trial. J Child Adolesc Psychopharmacol 2019;29(9):659–69.

75. Sanctuary MR, Kain JN, Chen SY, et al. Pilot study of probiotic/colostrum supplementation on gut function in children with autism and gastrointestinal symptoms. PLoS One 2019;14(1):e0210064.

76. Kang DW, Adams JB, Gregory AC, et al. Microbiota transfer therapy alters gut ecosystem and improves gastrointestinal and autism symptoms: an open-label study. Microbiome 2017;5(1):10.

77. Kang DW, Adams JB, Coleman DM, et al. Long-term benefit of microbiota transfer therapy on autism symptoms and gut microbiota. Sci Rep 2019;9(1):5821.

78. Sandler RH, Finegold SM, Bolte ER, et al. Short-term benefit from oral vancomycin treatment of regressive-onset autism. J Child Neurol 2000;15(7):429–35.

79. Bolte ER. Autism and Clostridium tetani. Med Hypotheses 1998;51(2):133–44.

80. Rodakis J. An n=1 case report of a child with autism improving on antibiotics and a father's quest to understand what it may mean. Microb Ecol Health Dis 2015;26: 26382.
81. Finegold SM, Summanen PH, Downes J, et al. Detection of *Clostridium perfringens* toxin genes in the gut microbiota of autistic children. Anaerobe 2017;45: 133–7.
82. Luna RA, Oezguen N, Balderas M, et al. Distinct microbiome-neuroimmune signatures correlate with functional abdominal pain in children with autism spectrum disorder. Cell Mol Gastroenterol Hepatol 2017;3(2):218–30.

The Impact of Applied Behavior Analysis to Address Mealtime Behaviors of Concern Among Individuals with Autism Spectrum Disorder

Benjamin Sarcia, MA, BCBA, LBA

KEYWORDS

- Inappropriate mealtime behavior • Avoidant restrictive food intake disorder
- Applied behavior analysis • Food selectivity • Food refusal • Liquid refusal • Autism
- Packing

KEY POINTS

- Applied behavioral analysis (ABA) is a mainstay of treatment in autism spectrum disorders (ASDs) for both core symptoms and noncore challenging behaviors.
- Feeding difficulties are common in individuals with ASD.
- ABA effectively addresses problematic mealtime behavior in children, and ample research exists supporting its use. The application in adults is not well studied.

INTRODUCTION TO APPLIED BEHAVIOR ANALYSIS

In 1968, Baer, Wolf, and Risley outlined the 7 dimensions of applied behavior analysis (ABA) in the first issue of the *Journal of Applied Behavior Analysis*. This article would become the seminal article of ABA and is still required reading in many graduate programs and course sequences in behavior analysis. Therefore, it is important to review these dimensions that have shaped the field of ABA and ultimately how intervention is provided to individuals with a diagnosis of autism spectrum disorder (ASD).[1]

The first dimension outlined by Baer, Wolf, and Risley is the applied dimension. This is the idea that an individual conducting applied research is doing so because the topic at hand is socially relevant. These authors provide the example of studying eating behavior in children who eat too little. This lends itself to the second dimension,

---

This article originally appeared in *Child and Adolescent Psychiatric Clinics*, Volume 29, Issue 3, July 2020.
Healthy Beginnings Feeding Therapy Program, Verbal Beginnings, LLC, 7090 Samuel Morse Drive, Suite 100, Columbia, MD 21046, USA
E-mail address: ben@verbalbeginnings.com

Psychiatr Clin N Am 44 (2021) 83–93
https://doi.org/10.1016/j.psc.2020.11.007
0193-953X/21/

which is that applied research must be behavioral. That is, the behaviors of interest are well defined, observable, and measurable, and the effect between the individual's behavior and the environment is established. When this effect is established and a functional relation proven between a behavior and a consequence, the criteria for meeting the dimension of analytical have occurred. This is what sets ABA apart from other disciplines. Establishing a functional relation indicates that when a specific event occurs or certain stimuli, such as items or people, are present or not present in the environment, a behavior will happen. On the contrary, such a relation may also indicate that when a specific event occurs or stimuli are present, a specific behavior stops or is inhibited.[1]

Behavior analytical procedures should be outlined in detail. These procedures are said to meet the dimension of being technological if they can be accurately replicated by an individual who is recreating the procedures and then achieves the same result as the original. This dimension is of great value, as behavior change procedures need to be replicated in order to be useful beyond the setting in which the original procedure was developed and assessed. Baer, Wolf, and Risely asserted that research reports be conceptually systematic in that they relate to the principles of ABA being addressed.[1]

For an intervention to be socially significant, it must be effective. This should go without saying. However, effectiveness is the sixth dimension of ABA. That is, a behavior change procedure must result in meaningful change that is observable by others. Coinciding with this is the dimension of generality. Behavior change following an intervention procedure should last as time passes. This change should also occur outside the setting in which the behavior change procedure occurred. It is important to note this, because clinicians should be planning for generalization from the beginning of a planned behavior change procedure in order to enact change that is meaningful to the individual, his or her family members, and his or her caregivers.[1]

APPLIED BEHAVIOR ANALYSIS AND AUTISM

Behavior analytical intervention among the ASD population has expanded considerably over the past five decades. This is due to intervention strategies being effective and reliable across many individuals. ABA is often used to address language deficits. For example, teaching an individual a functional communication response, such as a vocal request, sign, gesture, or picture exchange, is a common strategy for replacing problematic behaviors such as self-injury, aggression toward others, or property destruction. This is a common application in early intervention settings, but also among adolescents and even adults. Life skill development, such as tooth brushing or dressing, is another common application of ABA. For some individuals, this may entail systematic prompting, whereas others may learn from breaking down a skill into components and targeting 1 component at a time. Social functioning may also be a deficient skill area demonstrated by an individual with ASD. ABA has been utilized to develop behaviors such as sharing, turn taking, requesting play, and also more complex social behaviors such as asking a classmate to the school dance.[2]

APPLIED BEHAVIOR ANALYSIS AND MEALTIME BEHAVIOR

Defining features of a pediatric feeding disorder include: failure to consume enough food to sustain a healthy weight, or food that is developmentally or nutritionally appropriate, in addition to a failure to consume an age-typical variety of foods.[3] Malnutrition is often the result of these conditions going untreated, which can impact developmental growth. It has been reported by parents that hunger cues may be completely ignored by a child with feeding difficulties and that the child may go days without eating.[4] Frequently, these children will only eat food of a certain color or texture. Sometimes a specific utensil or plate is required for the child to consume the food presented to him or her.[5] Pediatric feeding disorders occur in developmental disorders, medical problems such as gastrointestinal conditions, or when there is a lack of exposure to a diverse variety of foods.[3]

Estimates of prevalence indicate that 30% of children with developmental delays[6] and as many as 90% of those with ASD[7] demonstrate some kind of feeding difficulty. However, it is important to note that approximately 45% of children who are considered to be developing typically exhibit inappropriate mealtime behavior (IMB) when novel food items are presented.[6] IMB refers to the individual engaging in behaviors such as covering his or her mouth, turning away from the bite, or pushing the bite away.

Medical problems can often cause a feeding disorder in infancy or childhood. Organic problems, such as gastroesophageal reflux disease (GERD), are reported as the most common medical problem associated with feeding disorders. Food refusal is often engendered by pain from medical conditions.[4] De Moor, Didden, and Korzilius found that in many children, problematic mealtime behaviors persist after the organic etiology of the feeding problem has been successfully treated (eg, medication used to control reflux).[8] These authors assert that early intervention is key to addressing IMB.

The Diagnostic and Statistical Manual of Mental Disorders, 5th Edition (DSM-5) terms feeding difficulties as avoidant restrictive food intake disorder (ARFID). Key features of this diagnosis include a feeding disturbance that results in significant weight loss, nutritional deficiency, and the need for supplemental nutrition. Additionally, this disturbance is not because of a lack of availability of food, a cultural practice (eg, religious fasting), medical condition, or specific eating disorders such as anorexia nervosa (AN) or bulimia nervosa (BN).[9]

A retrospective study of 98 children and adolescents found similarities between individuals with AN or BN and individuals with ARFID. Therefore, it was suggested that assessment and treatment should consider the overall health of an individual with ARFID because of the probability of concurrent medical complications as a result of the ARFID, whereas this is not true of individuals with AN or BN. However, data indicate that feeding issues may be the result of an anxiety disorder, obsessive compulsive disorder, or ASD. The result of this may be a nutritional deficiency that leads to medical issues.[10]

Among those with ASD, there may be no identifiable physical etiology for food refusal. It is common for children with ASD to engage in screaming, crying, disruption, and aggression when novel foods are offered. Given the nutritional concerns of poor dietary intake, it is common for growth to be impacted, as well as increased rates of constipation and disorders or diseases, such as diabetes, as the individual ages.[7] Poor nutrition and challenging behavior at mealtime can also impact the family dynamic. It has been found that when compared with typically developing peers, food-selective children with ASD are more likely to have a negative impact on their family overall, which includes spousal stress levels and the diets of other family members.[11]

The intent of this article is to provide an overview of common ABA interventions utilized to address challenging behavior at mealtime. Frequently, a quick solution to a complex problem is sought. However, this typically is not a reality, and thus the interventions described throughout this article have been empirically validated and are common practice by practitioners trained in ABA. For the purpose of this article, the terms feeding disorder, feeding difficulties, IMB, and food refusal will be used to refer to mealtime behavior that is not typical and of concern.

BASIC PRINCIPLES OF APPLIED BEHAVIOR ANALYSIS

ABA is a form of behavioral intervention extensively used in ASD. An ABA functional analysis would start with identifying the target behaviors to be changed. The behaviors would be specifically characterized. An analysis would be undertaken of the antecedents to the behavior (what preceded the behavior that could be instigating it) and consequences of the behavior (what occurred after the behavior that could be rewarding it). An intervention plan would be created, based on 3 core principles: reinforcement, extinction, and punishment. Reinforcement increases the frequency of a behavior. This is done by following the behavior with a preferred stimulus or reward (positive reinforcement), such as providing an individual with a piece of candy for picking up toys, or the removal of an aversive stimulus (negative reinforcement), for instance when one buckles his or her seatbelt and the chime stops sounding as a result of seatbelt buckling behavior.[10]

Extinction involves withholding the reinforcement when a specific, unwanted behavior occurs. That is, when this behavior occurs, the consequence maintaining the behavior is no longer delivered. As a result, the frequency of this behavior should decrease over time as the behavior is no longer being rewarded. For example, the child who has a tendency to call out in class no longer receives a response from the teacher. As a result, calling out behavior decreases, and the behavior of hand raising increases, as this is a more effective way to obtain the teacher's attention. Planned ignoring is a similar concept in which social reinforcers, such as attention or physical contact, are not provided for a period of time, after an undesired behavior has occurred.[12] These are often-used techniques in shaping mealtime behaviors.

Punishment consists of providing an aversive stimulus (positive punishment) or removal of a preferred stimulus (negative reinforcement) contingent upon a specific behavior. Contrary to reinforcement, punishment is always intended to reduce a behavior.[12] Punishment is less often utilized and never without first attempting reinforcement of more appropriate behaviors. The ethical code of the Behavior Analysis Certification Board mandates that options for reinforcement be exhausted prior to implementing a punishment contingency when intending to reduce inappropriate or potentially dangerous behaviors.[13]

ASSESSMENT

There is no standard for pretreatment assessment of a feeding disorder. However, common practice before implementation of an intervention typically involves a caregiver interview and observation of a meal, regardless of the discipline conducting the assessment. Behavioral assessment is a critical component for identification of factors maintaining IMB. Methods of this are described.

Descriptive assessment is a valuable tool for identifying factors that influence the occurrence of mealtime behavior. Borrero and colleagues describe conducting this type of assessment with caregivers in order evaluate the child's response to his or her caregiver, as opposed to an unfamiliar therapist. The benefit of this method is that it allows for observers to record the behaviors of the child and the parent, allowing for more accurate development of conditions for establishing baseline or conducting a functional analysis of IMB. However, descriptive assessment is not a proven method for predicting the function of IMB.[14]

In the field of ABA, functional analysis is considered the gold standard for determining the maintaining consequences of a behavior of interest. Iwata and colleagues developed a series of experimental conditions in order to identify contextual variables that resulted in the occurrence of self-injurious behavior.[15] In the case of feeding disorders, a functional analysis of IMB is often used to identify 3 functions: escape from demands to take bites, access to attention, or access to tangible items, such as toys, foods, or video.[16] For instance, if an individual is presented with a bite of novel food and the resulting consequence of IMB is removal of that food, the individual whose primary motivation is to escape this demand will engage in IMB most often in this condition. That is, the individual is sensitive to negative reinforcement, the removal of an aversive stimulus contingent upon a given behavior, which in this case would be the nonpreferred food.

Piazza and colleagues described their method of conducting functional analyses of IMB. After collecting descriptive information from parents, test conditions were developed based on this information. This included which novel foods to include in the assessment and the conditions to assess. For instance, if the parent reported that he or she never provided toys during meals, the condition to assess access to tangible items was not included as a part of the functional analysis, because this contingency was not occurring in the natural environment. The authors of this article were able to evaluate the function of their participants' IMB and develop a treatment package specific to this.[17] For instance, if it was identified that IMB was maintained by access to preferred toys, a component of treatment prescribed would be that the child only received specific, highly preferred toys when the child took a bite of the novel food being targeted in meal sessions.

INTERVENTION

In a review of 38 studies relating to food refusal and mealtime behavior among individuals with ASD and those considered be typically developing, Williams and colleagues found that 30 of these studies included reinforcement in at least 1 form. Twenty studies employed escape extinction as a strategy, while 11 utilized planned ignoring. Punishment was not listed as a strategy for any of these publications.[16]

Berth and colleagues explored the effectiveness of differential reinforcement (providing a toy and/or positive attention for acceptance of bites and drinks) and noncontingent reinforcement (access to preferred items regardless of mealtime behavior) among a sample of 5 children, all 5 years of age or younger and diagnosed with feeding difficulties. Three of these children had received a label of developmentally delayed, but ASD was not indicated for any of these children. A functional analysis of IMB was conducted for each child prior to treatment, allowing for the treatment package to be tailored to each child's specific mealtime behaviors of concern. These authors found that the provision of reinforcement when paired with escape extinction procedures was more often effective in increasing acceptance of bites and drinks than noncontingent access to reinforcement paired with escape extinction for 4 out of the 5 children.[18]

Reinforcement is frequently employed within a mealtime intervention package in order to increase the acceptance of bites and drinks. For instance, if the child accepts the bite into his or her mouth, he or she might receive access to attention and a preferred item for a specified amount of time. Reinforcement can be applied to various mealtime behaviors, such as chewing, swallowing bites and drinks, and using utensils. Sometimes reinforcement is provided regardless of behavior. This application is detailed further in this article.

Contingency contacting is a process in which reinforcement is maximized, and behaviors that serve an escape function are prevented. When employed specifically to feeding, these procedures involve provision of positive reinforcement for bites accepted and extinction procedures, such as blocking or planned ignoring when IMB occurred. A withdrawal design consists of removing the components of the intervention in an effort to assess behavior with baseline procedures in place and ultimately determine if the intervention is the reason for behavior change. It is expected that the withdrawal will result in a return to baseline levels of bite acceptance.[19] This is common practice within feeding intervention and can be a helpful practice to demonstrate to caregivers the importance of adhering to the mealtime protocol after discharge.

Reinforcement and extinction procedures are not only utilized to increase the acceptance of bites and drinks, but also to reduce the occurrence of expulsions. It is common for children to accept a bite or drink, access reinforcement, and then spit the food or drink out. Therefore, the child's treatment protocol has to be modified when this occurs in order to address expulsions. Coe and colleagues assessed the application of reinforcement and extinction in 2 children with food refusal. Neither child had a diagnosis of ASD. Nevertheless, this study was valuable in demonstrating that repeat presentation of expelled food was a necessary extinction strategy. That is, if the child spat out a bite, the feeder recovered the bite on the spoon and presented it to the child's lips again. This was done each time that an expulsion occurred. As a result, expulsion of bites was no longer a functional strategy for the child to escape taking bites. Reinforcement was also provided for swallowing bites, allowing for children to make progress in developing appropriate mealtime behaviors as the motivation for consuming the food was established by adding reinforcing items specific to each child.[20]

Within mealtime intervention, escape extinction is a fundamental treatment component. More commonly referred to as nonremoval of the spoon, this involves the feeder holding the spoon, bite, or cup to the child's lips until the child opens their mouth to accept the bite/drink or the time cap has been met. Note that a time cap is a predetermined meal duration. Other procedures related to escape extinction include presenting any bites/drinks that have been expelled again. If an expulsion of a bite were to occur, the feeder would collect the expelled food onto the spoon or obtain a new bite if this could not be done in a sanitary manner, and redeposit it into the child's mouth. This too would continue until the child swallowed the bite or the time cap was reached.[13 (AHEARN)]

An extinction burst is a common phenomenon when employing escape extinction procedures and is well documented in behavioral research. Cooper and colleagues[12] define an extinction burst as an initial increase in the frequency of a behavior when extinction procedures are implemented. Stated plainly, the individual may engage in more problem behaviors as the function of less frequent or lower-intensity behavior is not being served. In regard to mealtime behavior, an extinction burst may occur as the individual is attempting to escape taking the bite or drink and previously reinforced IMB is no longer effective. That is, the individual may engage in more IMB or higher-intensity IMB, necessitating that safeguards, such as padded seating or specific utensils be in place in order to manage the behavior safely while continuing to implement the intervention in an effective manner. In clinical practice, it is essential that caregivers be provided with an understanding of the extinction burst prior to intervention. This is important, because caregivers often exhibit an emotional response to the child's behavior and by discontinuing an intervention during the implementation of an extinction procedure would likely teach the child to engage in the increased frequency or intensity of problem behavior in order to escape any items perceived to be aversive.

As extinction is a fundamental element of behavioral treatment,[21] it is important to explore this principle further. Often times, treatments are not effective in increasing bite or drink acceptance, because the individual is able to gain escape from taking bites or drinks. Few studies have compared ABA intervention for mealtime behavior with other methods. One group conducted a comparison study of ABA to the Modified Sequential Oral Sensory Approach (M-SOS). Sequential Oral Sensory (SOS) is a popular mealtime intervention program that consists of an exposure hierarchy to food and drink, desensitization, and play. The SOS program does not employ the principles of ABA. The authors of this study emphasized that they were trained in the SOS via the workshops conducted by the creators of this approach and referred to their implementation within this study as modified, because certain modifications had to be made in order to scientifically evaluate the treatment. That is, they were careful to maintain the procedures as close as possible to the training and intervention materials that they had received as a part of this training, but modifications were necessary for data collection purposes.[22]

The comparison of ABA intervention to M-SOS is an important one, as M-SOS does not plan for extinction. The authors of this comparison study found that children in the M-SOS group did not make progress with accepting bites of food, although all were able to make progress to at least tolerate looking at novel food items. The children who had received ABA intervention demonstrated clinically significant improvements in bite acceptance and swallowing of bites. However, after the M-SOS program was completed, these children participated in ABA intervention, and all demonstrated clinically significant progress with the acceptance of novel foods. It is known that the key treatment component was escape extinction. In the M-SOS intervention, the child was able to control the reinforcer, which was access to escape. This was programmed for as a part of the ABA intervention; as a result, foods were added to each child's repertoire, because the child could not gain escape from taking bites.[22]

It is important to disclose that these findings were not without controversy. The authors were clear in reporting that they had received correspondence from the lawyers of the SOS program developers asserting that the desired outcomes of the program were not achieved because of systematic manipulations employed to evaluate the M-SOS treatment, such as specifically timed intervals for bite presentation.

Escape extinction was also investigated by Woods and Borrero. Of the 10 children evaluated, it was found that 4 children displayed behaviors consistent with an extinction burst when exposed to the escape extinction procedure. It was reported that all 10 children began accepting bites within 2 escape extinction sessions and that in cases where escape extinction is avoided or delayed, as many as 50 sessions have been required before the child has accepted a bite of novel food. This is significant given the time constraints involved in behavioral treatment of feeding difficulties. That is, it is common for insurance to authorize a predetermined number of sessions (eg, 40 sessions), and thus it is important to utilize that time with clinically effective procedures for addressing mealtime behavior. Additionally, these authors note that despite the effectiveness of escape extinction procedures, it continues to be best practice to implement this procedure in combination with reinforcement procedures, providing further support for the assertion that escape extinction is rarely effective on its own.[23]

Other strategies may be employed to increase the acceptance of bites. These are commonly referred to as antecedent strategies, as they occur before the intervention has commenced and thus before the child is engaging in IMB. Oftentimes these strategies are effective in reducing the intensity of an extinction burst and thus important to consider before beginning treatment. Ahearn assessed simultaneous presentation of preferred and novel food items to address food refusal in a boy with autism who refused all vegetables. This boy also was reported to have a profound intellectual disability. When ketchup was added to broccoli, corn, and carrots, the boy's acceptance of bites increased to 100%. It was reported by the child's teachers that following treatment, he began asking for these vegetables. The author does not explain if the use of ketchup was able to be faded out or if the ketchup was always necessary to promote vegetable consumption. It was also noted that elimination of 1 food group is considered to be a relatively mild feeding problem and that results of this strategy may not be the same for individuals who demonstrate more atypical eating habits at baseline.[24]

Packing is a common behavior that is exhibited by children with feeding disorders and entails the child accepting bites but holding the bites in their cheeks or on their tongue.[3] It is important to discuss strategies to address packing, because many children learn to accept bites, usually because reinforcement is provided for doing so; however, progress is inhibited by packing of these bites. That is, one would not continue to present bites to a child that has bites packed in their cheeks, as this would be a choking hazard. Levin and colleagues explored interventions for packing among 2 children with ASD. Both children were first evaluated by an interdisciplinary team prior to behavioral intervention in order to ensure that they were safe for oral feeding. For 1 child, offering purees and using a soft, rubber bristled brush, commonly referred to as a Nuk, was found to be an effective strategy for addressing the packing of bites. More specifically, a brush was used to remove the food from the child's mouth and then redistribute the food via the brush back on to the tongue in an attempt to facilitate swallowing of the bite. Reinforcement was also provided in the form of praise, contingent upon swallowing. This treatment package was effective in increasing swallowing of bites for this child.[25]

For some children, packing may be a chronic problem for which multiple strategies must be employed. For 1 child, Levin and colleagues found that escape extinction and redistribution of the packed bite were not effective when applied together. Therefore, other treatment components were added. This included a swallowing facilitation procedure, in which the feeder utilized the spoon to redeposit the bite onto the posterior area of the tongue while dragging the spoon along the tongue toward the entrance of the mouth. Eight cubic centimeters of water, a preferred drink, was also provided.[25] Although complex, this strategy was effective in decreasing the packing of bites and increasing swallowing for this child.

Although there are various strategies to address packing behavior, only recently was an assessment model developed to evaluate this behavior and guide treatment. Rivero and Borrero reported on a model that was utilized among 4 children with feeding difficulties, 2 of whom had a diagnosis of ASD. Some of the characteristics being tested included bite or bolus size, texture, effort, and food preference. These assessments were beneficial in identifying conditions in which low levels of packing occurred, enabling these clinicians to develop interventions related to the specific issues of the child. For instance, packing was found to be highest for 1 child when dime-sized bites of high-effort foods were presented.[26] Therefore, the authors suggest that an appropriate intervention would be to provide smaller bites of food that require less effort to chew and swallow. Although time- and labor-intensive, this evaluation procedure could be beneficial for identification of factors that influence packing, allowing for progress with treatment to occur, whereas progress may not have occurred otherwise. Additionally, there is benefit to caregivers in that the assessment results can be disseminated. That is, guidance related to the characteristics identified can be provided via caregiver training, perhaps ensuring that maintenance of gains made in treatment is more likely to occur once treatment is no longer occurring.

OUTCOMES

Unfortunately, publications assessing the long-term outcomes of behavioral treatment of mealtime behavior are few in number. Most often, parent report is provided in publications that detail outcomes of behavioral treatment for feeding difficulties. However, parent reporting often contains bias. Therefore, observation by a third party is needed to confirm the accuracy of parental report. Such observations are infrequently reported.

One report examined the outcomes children with autism treated with ABA for feeding difficulties in an inpatient facility. These authors divided those who responded into 2 categories. Of those within the 1- to 3-years postdischarge sample, 78% were reported to be consuming a greater variety of foods than they were prior to intervention. Additionally, refusal at mealtime had reduced for all but 1 participant, suggesting that the intensity and frequency of IMB had decreased. For those in the 3 or more years postdischarge sample, only 53.35% reported that acceptance of a greater variety of foods had maintained, while 3 caregivers reported that this area had become worse than it had been prior to intervention. However, it was reported that for all of these children, refusal at mealtime had improved. Therefore, this would suggest that if bite acceptance was decreasing in occurrence and IMB was not increasing, caregivers were no longer implementing the mealtime protocol, which would likely evoke IMB. When asked, 40% of caregivers indicated they were no longer using the mealtime protocol, compared with 28.5% in the 1- to 3-years postdischarge group.[27] Therefore, it is reasonable to believe that for children with ASD, a mealtime protocol may always be necessary to ensure that IMB remains low and bite acceptance maintains treatment levels. However, the implications for usage of a mealtime protocol throughout an individual's life are vague.

SUMMARY

Many ABA based interventions to address problematic mealtime behavior have been empirically validated and are considered to be best practice. Application of these interventions to a population with developmental delay typically does not require modification. However, information is limited as to what the long-term outcomes are for individuals who receive behavioral treatment and the implications for quality of life that these individuals have. Important questions relating to the maintenance of progress made in therapy and the overall health of these individuals have yet to be answered and reported.

Addressing feeding difficulties within the adult population with developmental disabilities also is an area that is, lacking. This is likely because of the limited intervention being provided to these individuals, given challenges such as being able to safely manage problem behavior that is predicted to occur when behavioral treatment utilizing escape extinction is implemented. This fact in itself suggests that the field of ABA should continue to explore strategies and intervention packages that are less likely to evoke an extinction burst when applied, while maintaining a high level of effectiveness.

DISCLOSURE

The author has nothing to disclose.

REFERENCES

1. Baer D, Wolf M, Risley T. Some current dimensions of applied behavior analysis. J Appl Behav Anal 1968;1:91–7.

2. Matson J, Turygin N, Beighley J, et al. Applied behavior analysis and in Autism spectrum disorders: recent developments, strengths, and pitfalls. Res Autism Spectr Disord 2012;6:144–50.

3. Shore B, Piazza C. Pediatric feeding disorders, Manual for the assessment and treatment of the behavior disorder of people with mental retardation. New York: Guilford; 1997. p. 65–89.

4. Piazza C. Feeding disorders and behavior: what have we learned? Develop Disabil 2008;14:174–81.

5. Schreck K, Williams K, Smith A. A comparison of eating behaviors between children with and without autism. J Autism Dev Disord 2004;33(4):433–9.

6. Ahearn W, Castine T, Nault K, et al. An assessment of food acceptance in children with autism or pervasive developmental disorders. J Autism Dev Disord 2001; 31(5):505–11.

7. Sharp W, Burrell T, Jaquess D. The Autism MEAL Plan: a parent-training curriculum to manage eating aversions and low intake among children with autism. Autism 2014;18(6):712–22.

8. De Moor J, Didden R, Korzilius H. Behavioural treatment of severe food refusal in five toddlers with developmental disabilities. Health Dev 2007;33(6):670–6.

9. American Psychiatric Association (APA). Diagnostic and statistical manual of mental disorders. 5th edition. Washington (DC: DSM-V; 2013.

10. Fisher M, Rosen D, Ornstein R, et al. Characteristics of avoidant/restrictive food intake disorder in children and adolescents: a "new disorder" in DSM-5. J Adolesc Health 2013;55:49–52.

11. Curtin C, Hubbard K, Anderson E, et al. Food selectivity, mealtime behavior problems, spousal stress, and family food choice in children with and without autism spectrum disorder. J Autism Dev Disord 2015;45:3308–15.

12. Cooper J, Heron T, Heward W. Applied behavior analysis. 2nd edition. Colombus (OH): Pearson; 2007.

13. Ahearn W, Kerwin M, Eicher P, et al. An alternating treatments comparison of two intensive interventions for food refusal. J Appl Behav Anal 1996;29(3):321–32.

14. Professional and ethical compliance code for behavior analysts. Behavior analysis certification board website. 2019. Available at: https://www.bacb.com/wp-content/uploads/BACB-Compliance-Code-english_190318.pdf. Accessed on November 1, 2019.

15. Borrero C, England J, Sarcia B, et al. A comparison of descriptive and functional analyses of inappropriate mealtime behavior. Behav Anal Pract 2016;9:364–79.

16. Piazza C, Fisher W, Brown K, et al. Functional analysis of inappropriate mealtime behaviors. J Appl Behav Anal 2003;36(2):187–204.

17. Iwata B, Dorsey M, Slifer K, et al. Toward a functional analysis of self-injury. J Appl Behav Anal 1994;27:197–209.

18. Williams K, Field D, Seiverling L. Food refusal in children: a review of the literature. Res Dev Disabil 2010;31(3):625–33.

19. Berth D, Bachmeyer M, Kirkwood C, et al. Noncontingent and differential reinforcement in the treatment of pediatric feeding problems. J Appl Behav Anal 2019;52(3):622–41.

20. Hoch T, Babbitt R, Coe D, et al. Contingency contacting: combining positive reinforcement and escape extinction procedures to treat persistent food refusal. Behav Modificiation 1994;18(1):106–28.

21. Coe D, Babbitt R, Williams K. Use of extinction and reinforcement to increase food consumption and reduce expulsion. J Appl Behav Anal 1997;30(3):581–3.

22. Peterson K, Piazza C, Volkert V. A comparison of modified sequential oral sensory approach to an applied behavior-analytic approach in the treatment of food selectivity in children with autism spectrum disorders. J Appl Behav Anal 2016; 49(3):1–27.
23. Woods J, Borrero C. Examining extinction bursts in the treatment of pediatric food refusal. Behav Interventions 2019;34:307–22.
24. Ahearn W. Using simultaneous presentation to increase vegetable consumption in a mildly selective child with autism. J Appl Behav Anal 2003;36(3):361–5.
25. Levin D, Volkert V, Piazza C. A multi-component treatment to reduce packing in children with feeding and autism spectrum disorders. Behav Modif 2014;38(6): 940–63.
26. Rivero A, Borrero C. Evaluation of empirical pretreatment assessments for developing treatments for packing in pediatric feeding disorders. Behav Anal Pract 2019;13:137–51.
27. Laud R, Girolami P, Boscoe J, et al. Treatment outcomes for severe feeding problems in children with autism spectrum disorder. Behav Modif 2009;33:520–36.

Assessment and Treatment of Emotion Regulation Impairment in Autism Spectrum Disorder Across the Life Span

Current State of the Science and Future Directions

Kelly B. Beck, PhD[a],*, Caitlin M. Conner, PhD[b], Kaitlyn E. Breitenfeldt, BS[c], Jessie B. Northrup, PhD[b], Susan W. White, PhD[d], Carla A. Mazefsky, PhD[b]

KEYWORDS

- Autism spectrum disorder • Emotion regulation • Reactivity • Assessment
- Treatment

KEY POINTS

- Research suggests that individuals with autism spectrum disorder (ASD) are more prone to have impaired emotion regulation (ER) than same-aged peers without ASD, beginning in early childhood and extending into adulthood.
- Cross-sectional research supports an association between impaired ER and more problem behaviors, aggression, co-occurring psychiatric diagnoses, and negative social outcomes in ASD.
- Broader and more sustained clinical impact may be achieved by focusing treatment on core ER impairments as opposed to a disorder-specific or problem-specific approach.

Continued

This article originally appeared in *Child and Adolescent Psychiatric Clinics*, Volume 29, Issue 3, July 2020.

[a] Department of Rehabilitation Science and Technology, University of Pittsburgh School of Health and Rehabilitation Sciences, 5036 Forbes Tower, 3600 Atwood Street, Pittsburgh, PA 15260, USA; [b] Department of Psychiatry, University of Pittsburgh School of Medicine, 3811 O'Hara Street, Webster Hall Suite 300, Pittsburgh, PA 15213, USA; [c] Department of Psychiatry, University of Pittsburgh School of Medicine, 3811 O'Hara Street, Webster Hall Suite 142M, Pittsburgh, PA 15213, USA; [d] Center for Youth Development and Intervention, Department of Psychology, University of Alabama, 200 Hackberry Lane 101 McMillan Building, Tuscaloosa, AL 35401, USA

* Corresponding author.

E-mail address: kellybeck@pitt.edu

Continued

- A multimodal assessment approach to ER measurement in ASD is recommended, with priority placed on measures and coding systems developed specifically for individuals with ASD.
- Although the research is in its infancy with small open pilot or waitlist control trials, existing research on ER in ASD suggests that ER can improve with treatment.

As eloquently summarized by Thompson,[1] emotion regulation (ER) is a complex, multi-faceted, and interactive process. Involving one's neurobiology, cognition, behavior, affect, and context, ER is the ability to monitor and modify arousal and reactivity to engage in adaptive behavior. ER involves intentional and automatic attempts to manage affect, as well as internal (acquired) and external (imposed by others) strategies.[1,2] Finally, ER is usually viewed functionally, meaning in relation to the degree that it is effective in facilitating goal attainment. In this review, we adopt a fully inclusive definition of ER that encompasses both reactivity (the speed and intensity of felt emotion) and the strategies (internal, external, intentional, automatic) applied to manage emotions.[3,4]

Although ER impairment in autism spectrum disorder (ASD) and its adverse influence on outcome has been acknowledged for several years (eg, Kanner's[5] mention of "disturbances of affective contact"), research on this phenomenon has been slow to develop. Herein, we offer readers a synthesis of extant research on both assessment and treatment of ER problems in ASD. This review is neither exhaustive nor is it an attempt to compare differential effectiveness of approaches. Rather, our goal is to summarize the advances made over the past decade with respect to assessment and treatment of ER problems in people with ASD across the life span. In so doing, we identify what appear to be the most promising ER measures for this population and consolidate the extant scientific literature on interventions targeting remediation of ER impairment. We focus exclusively on ER and not on the myriad of related problems (eg, anxiety, aggression). We also offer suggestions for research that must be addressed for the field to advance.

CLINICAL VALUE OF ADDRESSING EMOTION REGULATION IMPAIRMENT

A mother of a 9-year-old verbal boy with ASD and extreme emotion dysregulation wrote this of her son:

> My husband and I describe him as being at once the most capable and most disabled person we know; he can be the starting pitcher on his little league team without incident, participate and perform in a school-sponsored musical, all while not actually being capable of attending school (he is currently not at school at all, and is being referred by our local district for an out of placement evaluation). His dysregulation manifests in severe emotional outbursts, both verbal and physical; however, again, when regulated, he is more rationale, kind, and mature than his older neurotypical brothers…emotional dysregulation is absolutely his chief obstacle to living a full life and having the chance to enjoy his many talents (and they are many!).

This is, unfortunately, not an uncommon scenario. For many with autism, ER impairments are debilitating. As such, the top priorities for treatment trials identified by parents of young children with ASD are all related to problems regulating emotion (eg, distress, anxiety),[6] which is consistent with priorities identified by parents of older children and adults and adults with ASD themselves.[7] Indeed, people with ASD use psychiatric services at much higher rates than do individuals without ASD.[8]

Individuals with ASD may be predisposed to ER impairment due to differences in cognitive (executive functioning, abstraction, self-awareness) functioning, sensory sensitivities, and biological risks (**Fig. 1**) (see Ref.[9] for a more thorough discussion). Accumulating evidence suggests that ER impairment is more common, and more severe, for individuals with ASD than neurotypical peers.[10,11] Even in the first few years of life, children with ASD are less easily soothed and use fewer adaptive/constructive ER strategies as compared with same-aged neurotypical peers.[11] Although most neurotypical children learn to manage emotions enough to facilitate goal achievement by the time they reach school-age, many individuals with ASD struggle with ER impairments well into adolescence and adulthood.[9]

Impaired ER in ASD has been found to correlate with more problem behaviors (meltdowns, self-harm), co-occurring psychiatric diagnoses, and negative social outcomes for individuals with ASD.[12–15] Across the life span, ER impairment may present as aggression, more frequent and long-lasting negative emotions, and/or nervousness and social withdrawal.[7,16,17] In older ages especially, persistent rumination often days after an incident, intense reactions to social rejection, and continued reliance on parents or caregivers for calming (when no longer normative) is also commonly observed.[9,14,18] By adulthood, approximately 75% of adults with ASD in community samples have co-occurring diagnoses of either depression or anxiety, and ER impairment is believed to underlie these problems.[19]

Despite the varied manifestations of ER impairments in ASD and their presence across the life span, most psychosocial treatment research to address emotional problems has focused on children and the remediation of anxiety. These protocols generally do not address other common problems such as explosive behavior, meltdowns, irritability, anger, and depression. Although cognitive-behavioral therapy (CBT) has demonstrated potential for treating anxiety in children with ASD, response has been variable and effect sizes are lower than in youth without ASD.[20] Further, research suggests that these treatments are generally longer in duration than would be indicated for evidence-based therapies for similar conditions (eg, anxiety) in non-ASD populations, and that there is limited generalization of effects.[20] This suggests that it is important to try to remediate the causal processes.

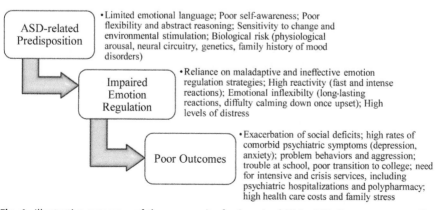

Fig. 1. Illustrative summary of the propensity for impaired ER in ASD, its common manifestations, and the resultant poor outcomes.

Broader and more sustained clinical impact may be achieved by focusing on core processes that underlie a range of problems, such as ER. Focusing on ER may facilitate effective treatment by addressing multiple behaviors and symptoms simultaneously. Further, ER impairments have been linked to lower parental quality of life,[21] suggesting that improving ER could have cascading positive benefits for the family system.

In sum, ER impairment underlies a variety of challenges faced by individuals with ASD and may present differently across the life span. For this reason, treatments that specifically address core ER impairments are likely to have a broader impact over a longer time horizon than treatments focused on secondary challenges arising from ER impairments (eg, behavioral problems in early childhood or anxiety in adolescence). Moreover, ER impairments are often cited as barriers to treatment focused on other ASD-related areas of need; thus, we recommend that (at least for some individuals) clinicians consider treating ER impairment before engaging in treatment for higher-level skills, such as social communication or social skills training.

EMOTION REGULATION MEASUREMENT IN AUTISM SPECTRUM DISORDER

The first step to improving ER is identifying it as an area of need. Screening to identify ER problems would be ideal to promote targeted prevention and treatment efforts. This is important, because although the ASD population as a whole is considered at high risk for ER impairment (as noted previously), there is wide variability. For example, even among psychiatric inpatients with ASD, there is a normal curve of ER severity.[22] Likewise, heterogeneity is considered a challenge within treatment contexts, with vast variability observed in response to even evidence-based ASD treatments.[23] Therefore, frequent measurement of progress is needed to evaluate how well an intervention is working for a particular patient and to inform whether a change in approach, dosage, or otherwise is needed. Finally, the establishment of new treatments as evidence-based is dependent on the availability of psychometrically sound measures that will be sensitive to treatment effects. Taken together, ER measurement provides the foundation for ER-focused treatment success.

Types of ER measurement methods include direct observation and behavior coding, physiologic monitoring, informant-report, and self-report questionnaires.[24] **Table 1** synthesizes the different ER measurement modalities, lists pros and cons to each modality, and references the most common measures used in ASD literature.

ER measurement in young children with ASD has often relied on direct observation and behavior coding. Thus far, naturalistic, frustrating tasks meant to elicit emotional reactions have been used, such as unsolvable puzzles and removing access to a desired toy.[11,17,44,45] Several researchers have applied coding systems to samples of children with ASD to characterize reactions (facial/bodily negativity, resignation, negative/non-negative vocalizations, coping strategies) to ER tasks.[11,17,45] However, the challenge with observational ER assessment in children with ASD is properly coding the expressed emotional reactivity, given atypical nonverbal communication and varying verbal capacity. Reactions may need to be coded in context of baseline communication skills, verbal capacity, and behaviors.[46] Achieving reliable coders is also time-intensive and not ideal for clinical contexts especially.

Physiologic measurement of ER is limited but has been used in several studies.[24] Respiratory Sinus Arrhythmia (RSA), a measure of heart rate variability, was used by several researchers to capture changes in heart rate during different tasks.[41–43] However, this has primarily been used to capture heart rate correlations to social competence and has only been secondarily considered as a possible peripheral marker of ER

Table 1
Measurement modalities and common measures to assess emotion regulation (ER) in autism spectrum disorder (ASD)

Method/Measure	ASD Studies that Used	Target Age
Self-report		
Pros: Feasible; Direct report from individual; Incorporation of patient perspectives is helpful for rapport		
Cons: Reporting of internal emotional states difficult for some with ASD; No measures validated in ASD; Not applicable to all with ASD (eg, with more severe co-occurring intellectual disability)		
1. Cognitive Emotion Regulation Questionnaire (CERQ[25])	Rieffe et al, 2011[18]; Bruggink et al[68], 2016	Adults Also a youth version used in Rieffe et al., 2011[18]
2. Difficulties in Emotion Regulation Scale (DERS[26])	Conner & White,[27] 2018; Maddox et al,[69] 2017; Swain et al,[70] 2015	Adults Also an adolescent version not previously used in ASD
3. Emotion Regulation Questionnaire (ERQ[28])	Samson et al,[71] 2012; Samson et al,[14] 2015; Cai et al,[10] 2018; Cai et al[72], 2019; Goldsmith & Kelley,[73] 2018	Adults Also a youth version Emotion Regulation Question for Children and Adolescents (ERQ-CA) not previously used with ASD
4. Response to Stress Questionnaire (RSQ[29])	Charlton et al,[74] 2019	Youth (developed on 11–19 y)
Parent-/Other-report		
Pros: Some options developed and validated in ASD (Emotion Dysregulation Inventory and Emotion Regulation and Social Skills Questionnaire only); Can capture concerns across contexts		
Cons: Finding a consistent informant may be difficult (especially for adults who may not live with caregivers); Limited to observable indicators of ER		
1. Child Behavior Checklist Emotion Dysregulation Index[30–32]	Samson et al, 2013; Samson et al,[14] 2015; Berkovits et al,[33] 2017; Keefer et al,[75] 2019; Joshi et al,[76] 2018	6–16 y
2. Emotion Dysregulation Inventory (EDI[3,22,34])	Mazefsky et al,[22] 2018; Mazefsky et al,[34] 2018; Conner et al,[35] 2019	6–18 y
3. Emotion Regulation and Social Skills Questionnaire (ERSSQ[36])	Butterworth et al,[37] 2014; Weiss et al,[38] 2018; Sofronoff et al,[77] 2017	Developed on 7–11 y

(continued on next page)

Table 1
(continued)

Method/Measure	ASD Studies that Used	Target Age
4. Emotion Regulation Checklist (ERC[39])	Scarpa & Reyes,[40] 2011; Berkovits et al,[33] 2017; Thomson et al,[78] 2015; Jahromi et al,[6] 2013	6–12 y
5. Response to Stress Questionnaire (RSQ[29])	Khor et al,[79] 2014; Mazefsky et al,[9] 2014; Conner White,[27] 2018; Charlton et al,[74] 2019	Developed on 11–19 y
Physiologic monitoring		
Pros: Biological measure, may be more objective		
Cons: Expensive equipment; Requires expertise		
1. Respiratory sinus arrythmia/heart rate	Bal et al,[41] 2010; Neuhaus et al,[42] 2014; Van Hecke et al,[43] 2009	Young child–adult
2. Skin conductance (electrodermal activity)	South et al,[80] 2012	11–16 y
Direct observation/behavior coding		
Pros: Can be done in naturalistic situations or in response to structured tasks; Can be done with young children		
Cons: Coding can be challenging due to atypical emotional expressiveness; Time-intensive to train coders and complete coding		
Observational tasks		
1. Laboratory Temperament Assessment Batter (Lab-TAB; Goldsmith et al,[81] 1999)	Jahromi et al,[11] 2012; Nuske et al,[44] 2017; Hirschler-Guttenberg et al,[45] 2015	2–10 y
2. Unsolvable puzzle task	Jahromi et al,[11] 2012	3–7 y
3. Affect regulation manipulation (toy removal)	Konstantareas & Stewart,[17] 2006	3–10 y
Coding systems		
1. Facial/body expressions (from Ekman & Friesen's Facial Action Coding System)	Jahromi et al,[11] 2012	3–7 y
2. Coping strategies/ER (from Eisenberg et al, 1996; Calkins et al, 1999)	Jahromi et al,[11] 2012	3–7 y
3. Engagement/Disengagement Coping strategies (from Grolnick et al, 1996)	Konstantareas & Stewart,[17] 2006; Nuske et al,[44] 2017; Hirschler-Guttenberg et al,[45] 2015	2–10 y

impairment.[42] Physiologic measures also typically require access to specialized sensors that can be expensive and thus are not regularly used in outpatient psychiatric care. However, an advantage of measures of physiologic arousal is that they can be used regardless of verbal ability, and emerging research has begun to explore how they can be applied to support clinical care. For example, Goodwin and colleagues[47] published promising proof of concept data on the use of physiologic data to predict imminent aggression onset, which may be effective in part due to its sensitivity to changes in overall arousal and reactivity.

Most research to date has used questionnaires to measure ER in individuals with ASD. ER assessment in school-aged children, adolescents, and adults typically consists of self-report and informant-report measures. This poses challenges given the limited psychometric research on the clinical utility of self-report ER measures in ASD samples, especially for individuals with limited verbal capacity.[46] This is complicated by inherent limitations in self-evaluation and awareness that is characteristic of ASD.[48,49] Further, informant-report assessment for adults with ASD are often not feasible or valid, especially for those who no longer live with parents. Thus, the options for ER measurement for adults with ASD are limited.

Researchers have primarily used existing parent-report assessments developed for general populations to assess ER.[6,33] The most commonly used informant-report assessments, typically completed by parents, include the Emotion Regulation Checklist (ERC)[39] and the Child Behavior Checklist (CBCL)[30,31] Emotion Dysregulation Index.[32] The ERC is a 24-item parent-report measure that includes 2 subscales: ER subscale (appropriate emotional expression, empathy, and emotional self-awareness) and lability/negativity subscale (inflexibility, rigidity, and dysregulated negative affect). The CBCL is a 113-item parent-report measure of psychiatric symptoms and behavioral functioning. Samson and colleagues[32] identified 18 items from the original CBCL that best characterize ER impairment, called the Emotion Dysregulation Index from the CBCL. In a study of 56 children, ages 6 to 16, they found greater ER impairment and severity than those without ASD.[32] The Emotion Regulation and Social Skills Questionnaire (ERSSQ) is an informant measure developed specifically for youth and adolescents with ASD.[36] The ERSSQ is a 27-item questionnaire with parent and teacher (25 item) versions to measure social skills that includes a few items on ER control.[37]

The Emotion Dysregulation Inventory (EDI) was specifically designed to measure ER impairments in youth and adolescents with ASD.[3,22,34] Mazefsky and colleagues[22] developed the EDI using the National Institutes of Health Patient-Reported Outcomes Measurement Information Systems (PROMIS) methodology. This 30-item scale was finalized using factor analysis and item response theory analyses using data from 1755 youth with ASD (aged 4–20) with normative data from a general sample of 1000 youth matched to the US census on age, gender, race, ethnicity, and region of the United States. The EDI is composed of 2 scales, Reactivity and Dysphoria. The Reactivity scale can be assessed using a 24-item long form or 7-item short form, and it measures intense, rapid, sustained, and poorly regulated negative emotional reactions, whereas the Dysphoria scale includes 6 items that capture withdrawal, minimal motivation and positive affect, and sadness or nervousness. The EDI has good reliability and validity, as well as superior discriminability to the ERC and CBCL Emotion Dysregulation Index, as well as others, in both ASD and general samples. Importantly, none of the final EDI items had evidence of differential item functioning (eg, psychometric biases) by gender, age, intellectual ability, or verbal ability, making it suitable for use across heterogeneous populations. Finally, the EDI has evidence of change sensitivity and offers clinical cutoffs for screening and interpretation. Young child (for ages 2 to 5 years) and self-report (for adolescents and adults) versions of the EDI are in development (R01 HD079512).

The most commonly used self-report ER measures in ASD samples include the Difficulties in Emotion Regulation Scale (DERS),[26] Emotion Regulation Questionnaire (ERQ),[28] and Responses to Stress Questionnaire (RSQ).[29] The DERS[28] is an adult self-report measure originally developed for individuals without ASD. It has 36 items that yields 6 subscales: nonacceptance of emotional responses, difficulties engaging in goal-directed behaviors, impulse control difficulties, lack of emotional awareness, limited access to ER strategies, and lack of emotional clarity. The ERQ consists of 10 self-report items that make up Reappraisal and Suppression subscales.[28] Although not initially conceptualized as a measure of ER strategies, the RSQ-social stress version[29] is a 57-item self-report and parent-report measure of coping strategies based on a 5-factor model of coping that categorizes ER/coping skills based on awareness engaging in the strategy and approach/avoidance of the emotion-eliciting stimuli (ie, involuntary engagement, involuntary disengagement, voluntary disengagement, primary voluntary coping, and secondary voluntary coping). Although several studies in ASD samples have reported satisfactory internal consistency and expected patterns of correlations with measures of related constructs (in support of concurrent validity),[13] none of these self-report measures were developed for ASD samples or have undergone thorough psychometric evaluation in ASD.

Ultimately, the research to establish the ideal means of measuring ER for individuals with ASD across the life span is in its infancy. The past 5 years has seen the application of newer coding systems[21] as well as the development of questionnaires (eg, EDI)[34] with promise for the assessment of ER in ASD. It is recommended that ER measurement consists of a multimodal assessment approach,[46,50] although much published research incorporates only one method of assessment.[24] For children, combining observational coding with interviews or informant-based assessment may be promising. Jahromi and colleagues[11] have developed coding systems specific to ASD in response to ER tasks that have been used in several studies.[51] For adolescents and adults, informant and self-report assessments may help to characterize ER impairments and improvements. Self-report ER measurement for individuals with ASD continues to be an area of need for future research, especially in transition-age and adult populations.

EMOTION REGULATION INTERVENTIONS ACROSS THE LIFE SPAN

Few interventions for very young children (preschool age or younger) with ASD include a component specifically aimed at improving ER, and none that we are aware of have measured change in ER as an outcome in a randomized control trial (RCT). The Social Communication, Emotional Regulation, and Transactional Support (SCERTS) model[52] explicitly teaches both self-regulatory skills and mutual regulation within the parent-child relationship. SCERTS takes a developmental approach that recognizes the interdependence between social communication and ER skills and integrates treatment in these domains. The only RCT of SCERTS reports improvements in social communication, adaptive behavior, social, and verbal skills with small to medium effect sizes in a group of 16-month-old to 20-month-old children with ASD; however, this study did not measure ER as an outcome.[53] Therefore, the efficacy of SCERTS for improving ER specifically is unknown.

The Joint Attention, Symbolic Play, Engagement and Regulation (JASPER)[54] model is another intervention aimed at very young children that includes a theoretic link to self-regulation. JASPER is a parent-mediated treatment focused primarily on sustaining periods of joint engagement and improving joint attention and play skills. The investigators point to the connection between joint attention and ER to argue that improvements in joint attention and joint engagement will lead to improvements in ER. One study using growth curve analysis reported decreasing child negativity (although this trend did not reach significance) and increasing maternal emotional scaffolding during the course of the intervention; however, no control group was included in the study and so the efficacy of JASPER for ER remains unclear.[51]

In contrast to very young children, several ER interventions are available for school-aged children (5–12 years). Attwood[55] and Sofronoff and colleagues[56–58] developed the Exploring Feelings, a CBT-based group intervention designed for children with ASD ages 9 to 12 with problematic anger. Exploring Feelings teaches emotion recognition and awareness through the use of cognitive restructuring, an emotional toolbox and thermometer, and strategy application. In an RCT with waitlist control (n = 45), parents reported that children in the intervention group showed a significant decrease in anger on the frustration and authority relations subscale of the Children's Inventory of Anger Parent.[58] Although this study did not use an ER measure, qualitative parent-report data showed that children receiving treatment reduced the number of anger outbursts and indicated that attending the sessions had been beneficial both for themselves and for their child.

Scarpa and Reyes[40] adapted the Exploring Feelings program for younger school-aged children (ages 5–7) experiencing problems with anger and ER, named the Stress and Anger Management Plan (STAMP). The STAMP program maintained the core components of Exploring Feelings with developmental adaptations appropriate for younger children (eg, shorter sessions, more games). Participants (n = 11) attended nine 1-h small group sessions while their parents attended a concurrent psychoeducation group. Pilot results indicated significant improvements of moderate to large effect in parent confidence in their child's ability to manage anger ($d = .63$) and anxiety ($d = .84$). STAMP participants also demonstrate large effects in improved negativity and lability ($d = .80$) on the ERC and significantly decreased frequency and duration of emotional outbursts. In a subsequent waitlist control study, 67% of STAMP participants (n = 18) were designated as treatment responders, based on significant changes in lability/negativity and a 20% decrease in the frequency, intensity, or duration of emotional outbursts.[59] Parents of STAMP participants also reported a significant increase in confidence of child's ability to manage anger.

The Secret Agent Society: Operation Regulation (SAS:OR) intervention targets ER in children with ASD through 10 sessions of manualized, individual CBT.[38] SAS:OR is based on the original Secret Agent Society, a social skills intervention designed for children with ASD.[60] SAS:OR was adapted to remove the social skills curriculum and replace it with ER (emotion awareness, mindfulness, acceptance) activities. This treatment also has a large focus on generalization of new ER skills to school and home environment through exposure activities and practice. Weiss and colleagues[38] conducted an RCT with a waitlist control on a sample of 68 children diagnosed with ASD. Moderate to large effect sizes of change were found over group and time in parent reports of ER skills (ERSSQ, $d = 0.79$; ERC, lability/negativity, $d = 0.58$), problem behaviors (BASC-2 Adaptive, $d = 0.71$).

The Intensive Outpatient Program for Emotion Regulation Treatment (IO-PERT)[61] is another ER treatment designed specifically for youth (8–12 years) with ASD and ER impairment. IO-PERT is the only ER treatment reviewed in this article that was designed for individuals with ASD and co-occurring Intellectual Disability. IO-PERT sessions occur twice weekly for 5 weeks and include both a child treatment group and a simultaneous caregiver education group. The treatment incorporates CBT, mindfulness principles, mediation practice, and Applied Behavioral Analysis techniques. Forty participants were enrolled in the IO-PERT treatment and 85% completed the intervention with high satisfaction. Statistically significant changes were found between pretreatment and posttreatment in psychiatric symptoms and behaviors measured with the CBCL and Aberrant Behavior Checklist (ABC). Clinical severity and improvement ratings measured by the Clinical Global Impression (CGI) found 53% of participants to be responders, 24% minimally improved, and 21% no change. Primary outcomes were evaluated with parent-report scales of behavior (CBCL and ABC), limiting conclusions on the specific ER treatment effects.

Relatively few interventions for adolescents or adults with ASD target ER. The Emotional Awareness and Skills Enhancement (EASE) program was developed to target impaired ER in adolescents and adults with ASD and measured changes in ER following an open trial directly using the EDI.[34,35] EASE aims to teach awareness of one's emotions and strategies to adaptively manage emotions by cultivating mindful awareness. Following increased awareness of internal emotional states, EASE participants learn cognitive skills (psychoeducation on thoughts, feelings, and behaviors, cognitive reappraisal, cognitive defusion), mindfulness-based distraction, and mindful breathing as a way to calm in heightened states of arousal. In an open pilot trial with 20 adolescents (12–17 years old) with ASD and IQ greater than 80, ER impairment, anxiety, and depression symptoms decreased with medium-to-large effect sizes. Participants and parents also indicated satisfaction with the intervention, including high ratings for helpfulness (M = 4.29 on 1–5 scale) and impact of the treatment in their lives (M = 4.18 on 1–5 scale). An RCT comparing EASE with individualized supportive therapy in adolescents and young adults with ASD and IQ >80 is ongoing.[62]

The Resourceful Adolescent Program–Autism Spectrum Disorder (RAP-A-ASD) is a school-based intervention intended to prevent depression symptoms in adolescents with ASD.[63,64] The intervention combines CBT and Interpersonal Therapy components for an 11-week individualized intervention. Although RAP-A-ASD does not specifically target or measure ER, there is 1 week, "Keeping calm" that focuses on ER by increasing awareness to physical reactions of emotions during times of stress. Mackay and colleagues[63] conducted an RCT (n = 29) evaluating the effects of RAP-A-ASD on depression, coping self-efficacy, and functioning. Parent reports of coping self-efficacy were significant at post (P = .023) and 6-month follow-up, but no change was found on depressive symptoms. Qualitative analyses suggested that 80% of participants reported improved capacity to manage emotions by remaining calm and being more flexible. Participants cited examples of less aggression, navigating social conflict better, and coping with rejection. Similarly, 63% of parents reported that the intervention enhanced ER and confidence, citing examples of participants feeling happier, more relaxed, and calmer.

In adults, Conner and White[27] adapted mindfulness-based cognitive therapy for young adults with ASD who have ER impairment in an open pilot study. Nine adults age 18 to 25 with ASD and ER impairment completed a 6-session individual therapy, where each session focused on teaching mindfulness meditations and targeted discussion and practice of one typically "adaptive" ER strategy and discussion of one typically "maladaptive" ER strategy, which were determined by client self-report on the RSQ. Self-reported improvements in DERS subscales for emotional awareness, impulse control, and access to ER strategies were observed, as well as decreased negative affect on the Positive and Negative Affect Scale.

Beck and colleagues[65] sought to establish feasibility of using Mindfulness-Based Stress Reduction (MBSR) with a group of adults diagnosed with ASD without adaptation to the standardized intervention. A sample of 12 adults aged 22 to 63 completed the 8-week group intervention (100% retention) with high levels of satisfaction and large estimates of effect in positive outlook ($d = 2.12$), satisfaction with life ($d = 1.08$), and mindfulness ($d = 1.10$). Although ER impairment was not directly measured in the feasibility trial, posttreatment qualitative interviews suggested that ER and increased awareness were candidate mechanisms of MBSR in this sample. Specifically, 60% of participants indicated that improvements in ER were the primary benefit experienced from the intervention, which has been found to be a primary mechanism of change in a variety of samples.[66]

Hartmann and colleagues[67] adapted Dialectical Behavior Therapy for adults with ASD in a small group study with 7 participants in which sessions targeted social communication challenges and ER impairment. The 12 group sessions included short mindfulness practices, identification of social situations that elicit emotional difficulties, and practicing social situations in session. Single-subject analyses on the 3-month group therapy indicated increased Social Cognition Index scores on the Social Responsiveness Scale-2 and ER improvement (decreased suppression and increased reappraisal on the ERQ) in most participants.[67]

Overall, the evidence for ER-focused interventions in ASD is quite limited. Nearly all existing studies are preliminary open trials with small sample sizes. The only randomized trials included waitlist controls rather than an active treatment comparison group. Some interventions include ER as a theoretic target mechanism, but they do not include measurement of ER as an outcome. Other than IO-PERT[61] and the interventions for young children, which to date have not measured effects on ER, most studies targeted children through adults who are verbal and/or have average cognitive ability. As such, the conclusions that can be drawn from the treatment research are limited. However, in general, the extant research suggests that ER can improve with treatment, with evidence for this from childhood (although not very early childhood yet) through adulthood.

SUMMARY

Nearly all ER research in ASD has occurred in the past decade. Although longitudinal studies to establish causation are lacking, the research overwhelmingly ties poor ER to a wide range of negative outcomes. This suggests that screening for ER impairment and the development and evaluation of ER-focused mechanistic treatments for individuals with ASD is an important direction for future research. Clinicians might consider focusing on treatment of ER as opposed to treatments for specific psychological symptoms or disorders. Further, treating ER impairment may be preferable before engaging in social skills training so that individuals can learn to manage emotions before engaging in stressful social demands.

Despite increasing appreciation of the importance of ER in ASD, treatment research for ER in ASD is in its infancy. The few clinical trials that have been done are preliminary in nature. For the most part, intervention studies have incorporated methods with efficacy outside of ASD, such as CBT and mindfulness, with promising results. This suggests that, in the absence of treatments with specific support of efficacy for ER in ASD, clinicians can use approaches to support ER outside of ASD with common modifications to support learning in ASD. It is also possible that approaches with efficacy for other treatment targets in ASD, such as CBT for anxiety or Functional Behavior Assessments and environmental supports for behavior, and so on, may be helpful for improving ER given that we know ER is strongly associated with these other concerns. However, measurement of ER outcomes is needed to better understand how other intervention approaches may impact ER.

Although there are very few measures that have been developed and validated for individuals with ASD, the recent development of 2 informant reports is promising.[24,46] More research is needed to develop sound self-report ER measures for adults with ASD. Although some studies have used biological indices such as measurement of RSA, this too, is in its infancy. Overall, the incorporation of technology into ER assessment in ASD has been very limited to date, although could be useful to consider more automated approaches to time-intensive forms of ER measurement, such as observational coding.

In sum, there is much to be done in terms of establishing empirically based approaches for ER assessment and treatment in ASD. More sophisticated clinical trials, such as sequential, multiple assignment, randomized trial (SMART) trial designs, integration of dissemination/implementation questions into trial designs, or comparison of multiple active treatments, may be useful to speed the state of the science. Although it may seem like a daunting amount of work remains to be done, we can continue steadfast with the potential for improved outcomes in mind. As stated by a parent of an adult woman with ASD, following initiating ER-focused treatment:

After 9 months of intensive sessions twice a week: results nothing short of miraculous. This, after trying every other type of therapy and medication out there. Without addressing her emotion regulation issues, nothing else was possible.

DISCLOSURE

This article was supported by DOD W81XWH-18-1-0284 (to C.A. Mazefsky) and R01 HD079512 (to C.A. Mazefsky). During the preparation of this article, J.B. Northrup received support through a T32 training grant from the National Institute of Mental Health (T32MH018269).

REFERENCES

1. Thompson RA. Emotion regulation: a theme in search of definition. Monogr Soc Res Child Dev 1994;59(2–3):25–52.
2. Gross JJ, Jazaieri H. Emotion, emotion regulation, and psychopathology: an affective science perspective. Clin Psychol Sci 2014;2(4):387–401.
3. Mazefsky CA, Yu L, Pilkonis P. The psychometric properties of the Emotion Dysregulation Inventory in a nationally representative sample of youth. J Clin Child Adolesc Psychol 2019. https://doi.org/10.1080/15374416.2019.1703710.
4. Zelkowitz RL, Cole DA. Measures of emotion reactivity and emotion regulation: convergent and discriminant validity. Pers Individ Dif 2016;102:123–32.
5. Kanner L. Autistic disturbances of affective contact. Nervous Child 1943;2(3): 217–50.
6. Jahromi LB, Bryce CI, Swanson J. The importance of self-regulation for the school and peer engagement of children with high-functioning autism. Res Autism Spectr Disord 2013;7(2):235–46.
7. Adamek L, Nichols S, Tetenbaum SP, et al. Individual temperament and problem behavior in children with autism spectrum disorders. Focus Autism Other Dev Disabl 2011;26(3):173–83.
8. Croen LA, Najjar DV, Ray GT, et al. A comparison of health care utilization and costs of children with and without autism spectrum disorders in a large group-model health plan. Pediatrics 2006;118(4):e1203–11.

9. Mazefsky CA, White SW. Emotion regulation: concepts and practice in autism spectrum disorder. Child Adolesc Psychiatr Clin N Am 2014;23(1):15–24.

10. Cai RY, Richdale AL, Uljarevic M, et al. Emotion regulation in autism spectrum disorder: where we are and where we need to go. Autism Res 2018;11(7):962–78.

11. Jahromi LB, Meek SE, Ober Reynolds S. Emotion regulation in the context of frustration in children with high functioning autism and their typical peers. J Child Psychol Psychiatry 2012;53(12):1250–8.

12. Guy L, Souders M, Bradstreet L, et al. Brief report: emotion regulation and respiratory sinus arrhythmia in autism spectrum disorder. J Autism Dev Disord 2014; 44(10):2614–20.

13. Mazefsky CA, Borue X, Day TN, et al. Emotion regulation patterns in adolescents with high-functioning autism spectrum disorder: comparison to typically developing adolescents and association with psychiatric symptoms. Autism Res 2014;7(3):344–54.

14. Samson AC, Hardan AY, Podell RW, et al. Emotion regulation in children and adolescents with autism spectrum disorder. Autism Res 2015;8(1):9–18.

15. Ting V, Weiss JA. Emotion regulation and parent co-regulation in children with autism spectrum disorder. J Autism Dev Disord 2017;47(3):680–9.

16. Giovagnoli G, Postorino V, Fatta LM, et al. Behavioral and emotional profile and parental stress in preschool children with autism spectrum disorder. Res Dev Disabil 2015;45:411–21.

17. Konstantareas MM, Stewart K. Affect regulation and temperament in children with autism spectrum disorder. J Autism Dev Disord 2006;36(2):143–54.

18. Rieffe C, De Bruine M, De Rooij M, et al. Approach and avoidant emotion regulation prevent depressive symptoms in children with an Autism Spectrum Disorder. Int J Dev Neurosci 2014;39:37–43.

19. Gotham K, Marvin A, Taylor J, et al. Characterizing the daily life, needs, and priorities of adults with autism spectrum disorder from Interactive Autism Network data. Autism 2015;19(7):794–804.

20. Kreslins A, Robertson AE, Melville C. The effectiveness of psychosocial interventions for anxiety in children and adolescents with autism spectrum disorder: a systematic review and meta-analysis. Child Adolesc Psychiatry Ment Health 2015;9(1):22.

21. Nuske HJ, Hedley D, Tseng CH, et al. Emotion regulation strategies in preschoolers with autism: associations with parent quality of life and family functioning. J Autism Dev Disord 2018;48(4):1287–300.

22. Mazefsky CA, Day TN, Siegel M, et al. Development of the emotion dysregulation inventory: a PROMIS.ing method for creating sensitive and unbiased questionnaires for autism spectrum disorder. J Autism Dev Disord 2018;48(11):3736–46.

23. Georgiades S, Szatmari P, Boyle M. Importance of studying heterogeneity in autism. Neuropsychiatry 2013;3(2):123–5.

24. Weiss JA, Thomson K, Chan L. A systematic literature review of emotion regulation measurement in individuals with autism spectrum disorder. Autism Res 2014; 7:629–48.

25. Garnefski N, Kraaij V, Spinhoven P. Negative life events, cognitive emotion regulation, and emotional problems. Pers Individ Dif 2001;30:1311–27.

26. Gratz KL, Roemer L. Multidimensional assessment of emotion regulation and dysregulation: development, factor structure, and initial validation of the difficulties in emotion regulation scale. J Psychopathol Behav Assess 2004;26(1):41–54.

27. Conner CM, White SW. Brief report: feasibility and preliminary efficacy of individual mindfulness therapy for adults with autism spectrum disorder. J Autism Dev Disord 2018;48(1):290–300.

28. Gross JJ, John OP. Individual differences in two emotion regulation processes: implications for affect, relationships, and well-being. J Pers Soc Psychol 2003; 85(2):348.

29. Connor-Smith JK, Compas BE, Wadsworth ME, et al. Responses to stress in adolescence: measurement of coping and involuntary stress responses. J Consult Clin Psychol 2000;68(6):976–92.

30. Achenbach TM, Rescorla LA. Manual for the ASEBA preschool forms and profiles. Burlington (VT): University of Vermont, Research center for children, youth, & families; 2000.

31. Achenbach TM, Rescorla L. Manual for the ASEBA school-age forms & profiles: an integrated system of multi-informant assessment. Burlington (VT): Aseba; 2001.

32. Samson AC, Phillips JM, Parker KJ, et al. Emotion dysregulation and the core features of autism spectrum disorder. J Autism Dev Disord 2014;44(7):1766–72.

33. Berkovits L, Eisenhower A, Blacher J. Emotion regulation in young children with autism spectrum disorders. J Autism Dev Disord 2017;47(1):68–79.

34. Mazefsky CA, Yu L, White SW, et al. The Emotion Dysregulation Inventory: psychometric properties and item response theory calibration in an autism spectrum disorder sample. Autism Res 2018;11:928–41.

35. Conner CM, White SW, Beck KB, et al. Improving emotion regulation ability in autism: the Emotional Awareness and Skills Enhancement (EASE) program. Autism 2019;23(5):1273–87.

36. Beaumont R, Sofronoff K. A multi component social skills intervention for children with Asperger syndrome: the Junior Detective Training Program. J Child Psychol Psychiatry 2008;49(7):743–53.

37. Butterworth TW, Hodge MA, Sofronoff K, et al. Validation of the emotion regulation and social skills questionnaire for young people with autism spectrum disorders. J Autism Dev Disord 2014;44(7):1535–45.

38. Weiss JA, Thomson K, Burnham Riosa P, et al. A randomized waitlist-controlled trial of cognitive behavior therapy to improve emotion regulation in children with autism. J Child Psychol Psychiatry 2018;59(11):1180–91.

39. Shields A, Cicchetti D. Emotion regulation among school-age children: the development and validation of a new criterion Q-sort scale. Dev Psychol 1997; 33(6):906.

40. Scarpa A, Reyes NM. Improving emotion regulation with CBT in young children with high functioning autism spectrum disorders: a pilot study. Behav Cogn Psychother 2011;39(4):495–500.

41. Bal E, Harden E, Lamb D, et al. Emotion recognition in children with autism spectrum disorders: relations to eye gaze and autonomic state. J Autism Dev Disord 2010;40(3):358–70.

42. Neuhaus M, Eakin EG, Straker L, et al. Reducing occupational sedentary time: a systematic review and meta-analysis of evidence on activity permissive workstations. Obes Rev 2014;15(10):822–38.

43. Van Hecke AV, Lebow J, Bal E, et al. Electroencephalogram and heart rate regulation to familiar and unfamiliar people in children with autism spectrum disorders. Child Dev 2009;80(4):1118–33.

44. Nuske HJ, Hedley D, Woollacott A, et al. Developmental delays in emotion regulation strategies in preschoolers with autism. Autism Res 2017;10(11):1808–22.

45. Hirschler Guttenberg Y, Golan O, Ostfeld Etzion S, et al. Mothering, fathering, and the regulation of negative and positive emotions in high-functioning preschoolers with autism spectrum disorder. J Child Psychol Psychiatry 2015;56(5):530–9.

46. Mazefsky CA, Herrington J, Siegel M, et al. The role of emotion regulation in autism spectrum disorder. J Am Acad Child Adolesc Psychiatry 2013;52(7): 679–88.

47. Goodwin MS, Mazefsky CA, Ioannidis S, et al. Predicting aggression to others in youth with autism using a wearable biosensor. Autism Res 2019;12(8):1286–96.

48. Hill E, Berthoz S, Frith U. Brief report: cognitive processing of own emotions in individuals with autistic spectrum disorder and in their relatives. J Autism Dev Disord 2004;34(2):229–35.

49. Mazefsky CA, Kao J, Oswald DP. Preliminary evidence suggesting caution in the use of psychiatric self-report measures with adolescents with high-functioning autism spectrum disorders. Res Autism Spectr Disord 2011;5(1):164–74.

50. Berking M, Wupperman P. Emotion regulation and mental health: recent findings, current challenges, and future directions. Curr Opin Psychiatry 2012;25(2):128–34.

51. Gulsrud AC, Jahromi LB, Kasari C. The co-regulation of emotions between mothers and their children with autism. J Autism Dev Disord 2010;40(2):227–37.

52. Prizant BM, Wetherby AM, Rubin E, et al. The SCERTS model: a comprehensive approach for children with autism spectrum disorders. Baltimore (MD): Brookes. Reichow, B., & Volkmar, F.; 2010.

53. Wetherby AM, Guthrie W, Woods J, et al. Parent-implemented social intervention for toddlers with autism: an RCT. Pediatrics 2014;134(6):1084–93.

54. Kasari C, Freeman S, Paparella T. Joint attention and symbolic play in young children with autism: a randomized controlled intervention study. J Child Psychol Psychiatry 2006;47(6):611–20.

55. Attwood T. Exploring feelings: cognitive behaviour therapy to manage anxiety. Arlington (TX): Future Horizons; 2004.

56. Sofronoff K, Attwood T. A cognitive behaviour therapy intervention for anxiety in children with Asperger's syndrome. Good Autism Practice 2003;4(1):2–8.

57. Sofronoff K, Attwood T, Hinton S. A randomised controlled trial of a CBT intervention for anxiety in children with Asperger syndrome. J Child Psychol Psychiatry 2005;46(11):1152–60.

58. Sofronoff K, Attwood T, Hinton S, et al. A randomized controlled trial of a cognitive behavioural intervention for anger management in children diagnosed with Asperger syndrome. J Autism Dev Disord 2007;37(7):1203–14.

59. Swain D, Murphy HG, Hassenfeldt TA, et al. Evaluating response to group CBT in young children with autism spectrum disorder. Cogn Behav Ther 2019;12. https://doi.org/10.1017/S1754470X19000011.

60. Beaumont R, Rotolone C, Sofronoff K. The Secret Agent Society social skills program for children with high functioning autism spectrum disorders: a comparison of two school variants. Psychol Sch 2015;52(4):390–402.

61. Shaffer RC, Wink LK, Ruberg J, et al. Emotion regulation intensive outpatient programming: development, feasibility , and acceptability. J Autism Dev Disord 2019;49(2):495–508.

62. Emotion Awareness and Skills Enhancement Program (EASE). ClinicalTrials.gov Identifier:NCT03432832. Available at: https://clinicaltrials.gov/ct2/show/NCT03432832?term=emotion+regulation&recrs=ab&cond=Autism&draw=4&rank=2, 2019, Accessed December 12, 2019.

63. Mackay BA, Shochet IM, Orr JA. A pilot randomised controlled trial of a school-based resilience intervention to prevent depressive symptoms for young

adolescents with autism spectrum disorder: a mixed methods analysis. J Autism Dev Disord 2017;47(11):3458–78.

64. Shochet IM, Saggers BR, Carrington SB, et al. The Cooperative Research Centre for Living with Autism (Autism CRC) conceptual model to promote mental health for adolescents with ASD. Clin Child Fam Psychol Rev 2016;19(2):94–116.

65. Beck KB, Greco VM, Terhorst L, et al. Mindfulness-based stress reduction for adults with autism spectrum disorder: feasibility and estimated effects. Mindfulness, 2020.

66. Gu J, Strauss C, Bond R, et al. How do mindfulness-based cognitive therapy and mindfulness-based stress reduction improve mental health and wellbeing? A systematic review and meta-analysis of meditation studies. Clin Psychol Rev 2015;37:1–12.

67. Hartmann K, Urbano MR, Raffaele CT, et al. Outcomes of an emotion regulation intervention group in young adults with autism spectrum disorder. Bull Menninger Clin 2019;83(3):259–77.

68. Bruggink A, Huisman S, Vuijk R, Kraaij V, Garnefski N. Cognitive emotion regulation, anxiety and depression in adults with autism spectrum disorder. Res Autism Spectr Disord 2016;22:34–44.

69. Maddox BB, Trubanova A, White SW. Untended wounds: non-suicidal self-injury in adults with autism spectrum disorder. Autism 2017;21(4):412–22.

70. Swain D, Scarpa A, White S, et al. Emotion dysregulation and anxiety in adults with ASD: Does social motivation play a role? J Autism Dev Disord 2015; 45(12):3971–7.

71. Samson AC, Huber O, Gross JJ. Emotion regulation in Asperger's syndrome and high-functioning autism. Emotion 2012;12(4):659–65.

72. Cai RY, Richdale AL, Dissanayake C, et al. Emotion regulation in autism: Reappraisal and suppression interactions. Autism 2019;23(3):737–49.

73. Goldsmith SF, Kelley E. Associations between emotion regulation and social impairment in children and adolescents with autism spectrum disorder. J Autism Dev Disord 2018;48(6):2164–73.

74. Charlton AS, Smith IC, Mazefsky CA, et al. The role of emotion regulation on co-occurring psychopathology in emerging adults with ASD. J Autism Dev Disord 2019;1–8.

75. Keefer A, Singh V, Kalb LG, et al. Investigating the factor structure of the child behavior checklist dysregulation profile in children and adolescents with autism spectrum disorder. Autism Res 2019;13:436–43.

76. Joshi G, Wozniak J, Fitzgerald M, et al. High risk for severe emotional dysregulation in psychiatrically referred youth with autism spectrum disorder: a controlled study. J Autism Dev Disord 2018;48:3101–15.

77. Sofronoff K, Silva J, Beaumont R. The secret agent society social-emotional skills program for children with a high-functioning autism spectrum disorder: a parent-directed trial. Focus Autism Other Dev Disabl 2017;32(1):55–70.

78. Thomson K, Riosa PB, Weiss JA. Brief report of preliminary outcomes of an emotion regulation intervention for children with autism spectrum disorder. J Autism Dev Disord 2015;45:3487–95.

79. Khor AS, Melvin GA, Reid SC, et al. Coping, daily hassles and behavior and emotional problems in adolescents with high-functioning autism / Asperger's disorder. J Autism Dev Disord 2014;44:593–608.

80. South M, Taylor KM, Newton T, et al. Psychophysiological and behavioral responses to a novel intruder threat task for children on the autism spectrum. J Autism Dev Disord 2017;47(12):3704–13.

81. Goldsmith HH, Reilly J, Lemery KS, et al. The laboratory assessment battery: Preschool version (LAB-TAB). Madison (WI): University of Wisconsin; 1999.

Sexuality and Gender Issues in Individuals with Autism Spectrum Disorder

Laura A. Pecora, BA, PGDip(Psych)[a], Merrilyn Hooley, PhD[a],
Laurie Sperry, PhD, BCBA-D[b], Gary B. Mesibov, PhD[c],
Mark A. Stokes, PhD[a],*

KEYWORDS

- Autism spectrum disorder • Autism • Sexuality • Sexual functioning • Relationships
- Gender • Transgender • Sexual orientation

KEY POINTS

- There is increasing awareness of the sexuality of individuals with autism spectrum disorder (ASD) and their interest in sexuality and intimate relationships.
- Core features of the condition render difficulties in attaining these. As such, individuals with ASD present with an increased risk of inappropriate sexual behaviors, unintentional sexual offending, and sexual victimization.
- Increased sexual and gender diversity among individuals with ASD has been noted. Different theoretic perspectives have been proposed to explain this, which include the possible influence of prenatal testosterone, and inflexible interpretations of gender roles that increase feelings of gender variance.
- Sex differences in sexuality domains have been observed, with females with ASD presenting with an increased risk of sexual victimization, including unwanted sexual experiences and contact than males with autism. Females with ASD also present with greater diversity in their sexuality, and are less likely to identify with their sex assigned at birth, and with a heterosexual sexual orientation than males with autism and typically developing females.
- Sex education programs that focus on developing sexual knowledge and skills required to attain healthy relationships and reduce sexual risks are effective, and therefore necessary for individuals across all levels of functioning.

This article originally appeared in *Child and Adolescent Psychiatric Clinics*, Volume 29, Issue 3, July 2020.
[a] Department of Psychology, Deakin University, 221 Burwood Highway, Burwood, Victoria 3125, Australia; [b] Department of Psychiatry and Behavioral Sciences, Division of General Psychiatry and Psychology, School of Medicine, Stanford University, 450 Jane Stanford Way, Stanford, CA 94305, USA; [c] Division TEACCH, School of Medicine, University of North Carolina, 321 S Columbia St, Chapel Hill, NC 27516, USA
* Corresponding author.
E-mail address: mark.stokes@deakin.edu.au

Psychiatr Clin N Am 44 (2021) 111–124
https://doi.org/10.1016/j.psc.2020.11.009
0193-953X/21/© 2020 Elsevier Inc. All rights reserved.

Sexuality in autism is now recognized as a normative, and integral aspect of development and functioning.[1,2] Existing research suggests that most individuals with autism spectrum disorder (ASD) display a clear interest in sexuality and relationships, and demonstrate a range of sexual behaviors.[3,4] However, the impairments in social skills and communication central to ASD potentially impact an autistic individual's expression and experience of sexuality by affecting their abilities to understand and interpret the social cues, emotions, and nonverbal behaviors of others.[3–5] Moreover, many individuals with ASD do not receive adequate, and developmentally appropriate sexual education,[4] and have less access to sexual health information from common sources than do their typically developing (TD) peers.[1,6,7] Sexuality-related problems often arise, with many individuals experiencing barriers in the development of a healthy sexuality and desired relationships. At times, these related challenges lead to vulnerability to abuse and/or contact with the criminal justice system.[8] Consequently, there are distinct differences in the sexuality and sexual functioning of individuals with ASD compared with the broader population.[3] Within this review, we present an exploration of the sexuality and gender issues of individuals with ASD and the implications for clinical practice and education.

SEXUAL BEHAVIOR

Sexual behavior involves a wide range of behaviors and activities with sexual or romantic intent.[9] Used to express and experience one's sexuality toward oneself or a partner, such behaviors include, but are not limited to, masturbation, kissing, oral sex, and sexual intercourse.[10] Studies investigating sexual behaviors within ASD consistently show that most individuals engage in solitary sexual behaviors. Masturbation is the most commonly reported form of sexual behavior, observed by caregivers (40%–77.8%), and self-reported by up to 94% of males across the entire range of the spectrum.[11–13] Levels of engagement in masturbation are similar between male adolescents with and without autism,[11,14] suggesting this to be a developmentally appropriate solitary sexual experience within this age group. Self-reported rates and frequencies of masturbation are lower among autistic females (20%–54.2%[4,15]), trending similarly to the rates in TD females (48.5%[16]).

Although most individuals with ASD engage in masturbation, some studies indicate substantially fewer report sexual behaviors with a partner. Within sexuality research, much of the literature notes that individuals with autism present with less lifetime sexual experience than healthy control subjects.[17,18] This has been evidenced by studies assessing self[18] and caregiver[2] reports, where adults with ASD report fewer sexual experiences, and less sociosexual behaviors than adults without ASD. The mean age of first sexual experiences is also up to 4 years higher among those with ASD (M = 18.7–22.1 years; SD = 2.7–5.9) than TD comparisons (17.6 years).[17,19] This has been attributed to a delay in the development of skills required to initiate sexual interactions, and a history of unsuccessful attempts at developing sexual relationships.[19]

However, other evidence suggests levels of sexual experience among high-functioning individuals with ASD that are comparable with that of TD peers.[14,20,21] In these studies, more than half of high-functioning participants reported some sexual experience, including intercourse.[15] Others have cited comparable levels of self-reported experiences of oral sex and sexual intercourse between ASD and TD groups.[11] Similarly, no differences in the breadth and strength of sexual behaviors have been observed between high-functioning individuals with ASD and non-ASD comparisons.[22] Thus, the current state of research suggests that although sexual experiences can be impaired for individuals with ASD across all levels of functioning,[17,18] some high-functioning individuals share similar levels of experience to TD peers. Although still in need of further exploration, differences in findings may be caused by the heterogeneous nature of the condition; the assessment of participants across variable levels of functioning; and the reliance on parental reports, which underestimate levels of sexual behavior.[14]

Inappropriate Sexual Behaviors

The social and communication deficits typical to autism often interfere with abilities to establish and maintain peer networks. As a result, individuals with ASD have fewer social sources, and thus fewer opportunities to acquire social wisdom in relation to sexuality and sexual health.[7] When low levels of sexual knowledge are combined with an expressed desire to facilitate meaningful relationships,[23] some authors suggest that individuals with ASD lack the understanding and skills required to initiate these relationships in a healthy way.[7,24] Because individuals with ASD also experience difficulties discriminating between the behaviors that are considered appropriate across different settings,[7,24] they may naively engage in inappropriate courting behaviors as a means of seeking contact, or initiating relationships with others.[7,24,25] Consequently, the risk of individuals with ASD pursuing potential partners in ways construed as threatening (eg, engaging in inappropriate touching, stalking) is higher than in TD peers.[7,26]

Other core features of ASD can impact sexuality. Restricted and repetitive behaviors and stereotyped interests can manifest as a preoccupation with specific sexualized behaviors, particularly in adulthood.[5] Sensory sensitivities can also impact sexual experiences, with some hypersensitive individuals experiencing soft physical touches as unpleasant.[5] Others experience an underreaction to sensory stimuli, and require above-average stimulation to become sexually aroused.[5] Lack of awareness of the behaviors that are considered appropriate in public settings[2,27] can lead to expression of sexuality in socially unacceptable ways.[20] As such, individuals with ASD present with an increased risk of engaging in hypersexual, or problematic sexual behaviors.[5,28] Some evidence of this comes from cases of public, or deviant masturbation, which includes compulsive masturbation and the use of peculiar masturbation techniques.[12,29]

Sexual problems can also arise, with cited instances of unwanted attempts at intercourse, paraphilic sexual fantasies,[5,28] pedophilia, and fetishism,[5,12] particularly in males. Although problematic behaviors have been observed in individuals across all levels of functioning,[5] the occurrence and frequency of hypersexual behaviors has been associated with greater levels of autism symptoms.[30]

Because inappropriate courting and problematic sexual behaviors are recognized as forms of sexual offending, individuals with ASD face increased risks of coming into contact with the criminal justice systems.[8] Consequently, there is a higher prevalence of individuals with ASD who have been charged with sexual offending for the naive engagement in inappropriate behaviors. Evidence of unintentional sexual offending has been drawn from case studies, citing sexual preoccupations with the genitalia of others,[31] inappropriate sexual contact with minors,[32] and indirect sexual assaults in high-functioning males.[33] Quantitative investigations have likewise identified an overrepresentation of ASD cases in forensic settings.[24] These studies have identified links between obsessional interests around sexuality, heightened social naivety, and an increased prevalence of sexual offending in the form of sexually abusive and paraphilic behaviors; indecent exposure; and public masturbation.[13,24] It is essential that the criminal justice system consider how characteristics of autism are involved in the commission of a sexual offense. Such offenses that are sexually deviant in their expression may be a paraphilia or may be the pursuit of deep interests, or sensory seeking behavior that co-occurs with a sexual behavior. This phenomenon has been referred to as "counterfeit deviance."[34] Counterfeit deviance may manifest itself in the form of people using objects to enable them to masturbate more easily because of motor challenges. It may be that a noneroticized object has been incorporated into a routine, it may be lack of access to more traditional lubricants or a sensory preference.[28] Van Bourgondien and colleagues[13] describe multiple instances of people with autism incorporating common household items (shampoo bottles, suitcases, books) into their masturbation routines.

Viewing images of child exploitation is, unfortunately, an increasing point of contact with the criminal justice system for people on the autism spectrum. In his excellent piece, *Asperger's Syndrome and the Criminal Law: The Special Case of Child Pornography*,[35] criminal defense attorney Mark Mahoney explores the characteristics of autism that may result in this particular offense. Unemployment and underemployment often result in unfettered free time to spend online. Compounded by a desire for social interaction and intimate relationships that is foiled by social anxiety and isolation and further exacerbated by absent or inadequate sexuality education, a perfect recipe for disaster has been created. Difficulty reading facial expressions and impairments in Theory of Mind may make it difficult for people with autism to read the expressions of distress on the faces of the children in the images or video and further impair their ability to consider how their behavior creates a market for further exploitation of children. The mainstream sexualization of children may create a stimulus equivalence from a behavior analytical perspective wherein the person with autism responds to an image of a sexualized minor in the same way they would respond to the sexualized image of an adult.[36] Finally, deficits in executive functioning may compromise a person's ability to think through the consequences of being apprehended. They may be unaware or unable to think through the lifetime consequences of being arrested, going to prison, and being placed on a sex offender registry.[37,38]

Because individuals who commit sexual offences often do so in the context of their autism symptoms,[37] these cases highlight the complexities around the ways criminal justice systems should respond to these sexual offences. Moreover, qualitative research highlights that the negative outcomes that commonly occur following criminal charges are exacerbated among individuals with ASD, who do not have their developmental needs met, and are often subject to isolation and victimization when placed in the prison system.[8,39] Thus, the reviewed studies highlight the innate vulnerabilities of individuals with ASD that increase the risk of being charged with sexual offences. They also support the requirements of criminal justice, and education systems to recognize, and aim to reduce these.[8]

SEXUAL VICTIMIZATION

Studies investigating sexual experiences within ASD have identified an increased risk of sexual victimization and abuse.[23,40,41] Much of the literature documenting cases of sexual victimization has been drawn from child and adolescent samples.[40,42] Within all reviewed studies, significantly higher rates of sexual abuse (16.6%)[40] and coercive sexual victimization[42] have been observed among youth with ASD than among the broader population (11.5%[43]). Among adults, those with ASD are between two and three times more likely to have experienced sexual victimization in the form of sexual coercion,[23] unwanted sexual contact[23,25,44] or sexual experiences,[41] and rape[23,25] than non-ASD control subjects. Similar patterns have also been observed in female-only samples, with one study identifying an increased proportion of lifetime instances of sexual abuse, and unwanted sexual touching among females with ASD (62%) than non-ASD females (53%).[45] Although these rates are striking, an additional concern is that the communication impairments prevalent in ASD make individuals less likely to identify and report these experiences as forms of sexual victimization.[46,47] Because cases of sexual victimization are often underreported by individuals with ASD,[48] and in research contexts,[45] it is likely that the rates observed in these studies are underestimates.

Sex differences have also been observed in sexual victimization, with females with ASD presenting with an increased risk of adverse sexual experiences, including regretted, and unwanted sexual experiences, than male counterparts.[41] Qualitative studies have identified a host of sexual vulnerabilities that although not unique, are increased among females with ASD. Some documented cases include the naive engagement in promiscuity as a means of initiating desired relationships,[29,49] and poor choices of abusive romantic partners.[50] Others have cited an increased susceptibility to sexual exploitation because of being overly trusting, and more likely to misinterpret the sexual intentions of others.[51] Levels of autistic traits have also been associated with risk to sexual abuse, where females with higher levels of ASD symptoms being likely to have been sexually abused (40.1% vs 26.7%), or experience being pressured into sexual contact (25.4% vs 15.6%) compared with females with lower levels of autistic traits.[52]

Sexual orientation within autism is also an important factor. Evidence from Pecora and colleagues[53] suggested that homosexual females with ASD were more vulnerable to regretted, and unwanted sexual behavior compared with their heterosexual ASD counterparts. Because females with ASD[17,54] and those within a sexual minority also present with higher rates of internalizing conditions, such as isolation, anxiety, and depressed mood states,[55,56] it is possible that the psychological impact of sexual victimization, together with identifying as within these minority groups, may be exacerbated among homosexual females with ASD.

The same mechanisms that underlie increased risk of offending may also serve an explanatory role in the heightened risks for sexual victimization. These include deficits in social understanding, communication difficulties, and impaired theory of mind.[47] These characteristics are associated with difficulty interpreting the intentions of others, and thus difficulty discriminating between safe and unsafe individuals and situations.[45,57,58] Individuals with ASD are also less able to recognize the deceptive emotions of others,[54] or detect violations in social exchange rules.[52] As such, they are less likely to make accurate character judgements of potential offenders who approach them.[42] The impact of these deficits is often exacerbated by a lack of sexual knowledge,[23] which limits understanding of ways to protect themselves from unsafe situations and risky sexual practices. Difficulties building interpersonal relationships, and thus fewer protective peer networks, can also act as risk factors for sexual abuse.[47,59] Finally, the social and emotional challenges related to ASD may increase the vulnerability of individuals to be viewed as easy targets of sexual abuse by opportunistic offenders.[57] Consequently, the key features of ASD seem to act as a predictable set of risk factors for sexual victimization and abuse.

SEXUAL ORIENTATION

Sexual orientation is a multidimensional construct comprising the domains of sexual identity, sexual interests, sexual attraction, and sexual contact.[9,22] Each domain is distinct from one another. Each influences an individual's underlying sexual preference toward others.[18] There is a considerable body of research citing a higher prevalence of nonheterosexual orientations in ASD than in the general population.[2,12,29,60–62]

Initial observations of this increased prevalence were drawn from caregivers reports of low functioning males, where up to 40% of residents reported nonheterosexual orientations.[12,13] More recently, self-report studies assessing aspects of sexuality have observed similar patterns, where adolescents and adults with ASD reported lower levels of heterosexual interests, behaviors, and orientation (30.3%–50.6%) than non-ASD control subjects (69.7%–90.4%).[2,22,60–62] Higher rates of same-sex and bisexual interests and attraction were also observed in these studies, in addition to greater feelings of asexuality than TD groups.

In all reviewed studies, these trends were more apparent for females, who expressed more attraction to individuals of the same, or both sexes than males with ASD. Others have observed increased sexual diversity in females with ASD, yet similar proportions (5%–10%) of same sex attraction and experience between males with and without ASD.[19,30] Despite this, males with ASD have also been found to report more tolerant attitudes toward same sex sexuality and behavior than adolescent peers without ASD.[11]

Greater diversity in sexual orientation has also been reported in studies assessing female-only samples, where females with ASD have been more likely to identify as nonheterosexual than TD control subjects.[45,53] Although greater identification with a homosexual sexual orientation has been reported by one empirical study,[53] several research papers have noted that females with ASD are between three and four times more likely to identify as bisexual than females without ASD.[19,53] Similarly, proportions of females with ASD identifying with a sexual minority (92%) were also larger than among non-ASD females (72%), despite unexpectedly high rates of sexual minority status in Bush's[45] comparison sample.

GENDER IDENTITY

There is evidence that individuals with ASD present with more diverse gender identities than the broader population. Gender identity refers to the self-identified gender conception of oneself,[63] the breadth of gender nouns is considerably greater than male, female, or transgender (see Ref.[64] for a listing). When there is incongruence between an individuals' gender identity and biologic sex, an individual may identify along a spectrum of a gender identity.[65,66] An individual's gender identity is also associated with the cultural and societal roles, behaviors, and attitudes that are considered typical for individuals based on their biologic sex.[63,67]

Gender Variance

Gender variance (GV) is a term used to describe an individual's variation in gender role and typical behaviors, which deviate from culturally specific gender norms.[67] Because GV is not associated with feelings of distress, it is distinct from gender dysphoria (GD).[67] Increasingly clinical[68] and quantitative findings[69,70] suggest a relationship between ASD and GV. Within child and adolescent samples, individuals with ASD are between 7.59[63] and 7.76[70] times more likely to express feelings of GV than TD control subjects. Collapsed across age, an increased prevalence of GV has also been observed in ASD,[69] where 5.2% of males, and 7.2% of females with ASD have expressed feelings of GV. Although gender effects were not found in this study, the observed rates were significantly higher than the 0.7% reported in the general population. Similar patterns have also been observed in adults, where GV has been expressed by 11.3% of adults with ASD, yet 5% of TD control subjects.[71] These findings are consistent with other studies of adults with ASD, which show greater diversity in gender identity than healthy control subjects.[51,60] For example, George and

Stokes[60] found that rates of transgender identity (3.9%) were at least 20 times higher among adults with ASD than census-based prevalence estimates in the broader population. Within female-specific research, females with ASD are also more likely to identify as transgender,[52] or with a more fluid gender identity[45] than individuals without ASD assigned female at birth. Similarly, females with ASD are also more likely to report masculinized gender behaviors in childhood, and a more masculinized gender identity than same-sex control subjects.[19] Although studies examining ASD and GV exclusive from GD are limited, these emerging findings contribute to growing bodies of literature suggesting a co-occurrence of ASD and increased gender diversity overall.

Gender Dysphoria

Various studies have reported an overlap between ASD and GD. Within the Diagnostic and Statistical Manual of Mental Disorders-5,[72] GD refers to significant levels of distress, which result from the incongruence between one's birth-assigned gender and one's experienced gender. This is also experienced with a persistent and strong desire to be of another gender.[73] Within clinical settings, there has been an increasing number of descriptions of gender-related concerns in individuals who fulfill diagnostic criteria for ASD. Numerous case studies have described evidence of GD in ASD patients,[73–75] and cases of co-occurring GD and ASD diagnoses.[76,77] An increased prevalence of GD characteristics in ASD has also been identified,[60] with a recent study observing higher scores on measures of GD traits in adults with ASD than TD control subjects.

Other approaches have examined rates of ASD symptoms in individuals referred to gender identity clinics. Findings of a systematic study identified an overrepresentation of ASD diagnoses in a sample of 204 children (6.4%) and adolescents (9.4%) referred for GD.[78] This incidence is significantly higher than the global prevalence of ASD, which ranges from 1% to 2%.[79] In another study that assessed the presence of various domains of autistic traits using the Children's Social Behavior Questionnaire,[80] children and adolescents with GD demonstrated greater levels of autistic-like characteristics than TD comparisons.[81] Levels of autistic traits in the GD group were, however, lower than children and adolescents with an ASD diagnosis.

Additional studies have used Baron-Cohen's[82] Autism Quotient (AQ) to quantify levels of autistic traits in GD participants. Examining the co-occurrence of autistic traits in adults with GD, Bejerot and Eriksson[19] found GD participants scored higher on the AQ than TD comparisons. Pasterski and colleagues[83] also cited evidence of this association, where 4.8% of males and 7.1% of females with GD met the cutoff score for screening diagnosis (AQ >32). Another study[84] found females with GD yielded higher AQ scores than TD females. However, differences in AQ scores between transgender males and males that identified with their sex at birth were not significant. Together, these studies suggest that GD individuals present with greater clinically significant ASD symptoms than those in the general population.

Sex Differences

Within reviewed studies, sex differences in rates of GV and GD have been found between males and females with ASD.[3,59,85] Although limited in number, studies assessing participants according to their biologic sex have identified elevated rates of GV and gender-nonconforming feelings in females (22%) than in males with ASD (8%).[3] This is further supported by a recent study using an adult population,[55] which found that females with ASD presented with greater levels of gender dysphoric traits than male counterparts. Similarly, levels of clinically significant ASD symptoms in GD samples have been higher among those assigned a female sex at birth.[85] Thus, the overlap between ASD and gender-related issues seem to be most apparent for females in this group.

GENDER AND SEXUAL DIVERSITY: UNDERLYING EXPLANATIONS

Various hypotheses have been proposed to explain the increased gender and sexual diversity among individuals with autism. Neurobiologic theories point to the influence of increased exposure to fetal testosterone, and its links with autistic traits, and neural masculinization.[86] Prenatal exposure to testosterone has been associated with an increased development of male-based traits, behaviors, and sexual preferences, particularly in females with ASD.[83,86] However, the fetal testosterone theory would only suggest variation in gender and sexual identity in females, and thus does not explain the links between ASD and sexual diversity among males with ASD. However, this would only suggest a link between GD and women with autism, but does not go toward explaining the link between GD and autistic traits also found among males.

Psychosocial theories suggest that the key features of ASD, including stereotyped interests and cognitive rigidity, contribute to inflexible stereotypical beliefs about gender roles.[81] This hypothesis postulates that individuals with ASD may not reach the level of cognitive flexibility required to understand that gender roles can vary outside gender stereotypes.[78,81] Thus, they may be more prone to develop a trans-gender identity if interests and characteristics do not fit these stereotypes.[71,78,81] Another possible explanation is that because of limited opportunities to meet and develop relationships with others, and less awareness of social norms, an individual's birth sex may not be relevant when choosing sexual or romantic partners.[22,81] This may therefore account for increased fluidity around sexual preferences observed in ASD.[45,62] Although further exploration into the mechanisms driving gender and sexual diversity within ASD is required, current models propose a multivariate account, where an interaction of all possible influences, rather than a single factor, provides a more accurate explanation for these findings.[81]

CLINICAL IMPLICATIONS

It is important to recognize that impairments in the social and communication domains of functioning, together with a lack of sexually appropriate education, and a desire for a romantic or sexual relationship are contributing to the range of problematic sexual behaviors identified in this review. Not all individuals with ASD express problematic sexual behaviors. The identified challenges experienced by individuals with ASD reflect the inherent need for developmentally appropriate sexual education with an emphasis on the underlying social competencies required for developing healthy intimate relationships tailored to the unique needs of each patient. Clinicians may consider evidence-based relationship education, such as that offered by the PEERS for young adults,[87] Sexuality Education for Youth on the Autism Spectrum,[88] or Tackling Teenage programs,[89] which demonstrate success. Likewise, social skills training, which in the form of social stories or video modeling can assist in teaching appropriate behaviors in social situations, and ways to interact with potential romantic or sexual partners.[26,90] Because social stories have also been successful in reducing disruptive behaviors,[90,91] they could perhaps be applied to target and decrease inappropriate sexual behaviors.

Professionals should likewise be attuned to recognize the risk factors, warning signs, and symptoms of potential sexual offending and sexual victimization, and previous unwanted sexual experiences within clients with ASD. Tailored support programs would benefit from greater understanding of the factors that are related to increased sexual risks particularly among females with ASD, and the negative psychological and health consequences that are associated with experiences of victimization.[92] Therapeutic techniques including assertiveness training, which have successfully reduced risks of sexual victimization in TD groups,[93] can also enhance personal control over future instances of potential victimization. Thus, educational efforts would strengthen the personal skills required to make safe and positive decisions in sexual situations, and promote the sexual health and well-being of individuals with ASD overall.

In a clinical setting, awareness of the different expressions of sexuality and increased sexual and gender diversity in ASD is necessary. Thus, clinicians should provide opportunities to share the concerns that surround the development and expression of a healthy sexuality, and fulfilling sexual identity. Individuals with ASD and those who identify with a sexual minority experience sexuality-related challenges and have unique health care needs.[55,94] These include poor mental health and well-being in relation to minority stress,[55,94] complex socioemotional problems,[55,93] and increased vulnerabilities to sexual victimization.[52,95] It is therefore important for professionals to be aware of these, particularly among individuals with autism who identify with a gender or sexual minority. Through increased understanding, this knowledge can also be used to develop strategies and services that aim to provide individuals with ASD the skills required to develop a fulfilling gender and sexual identity, and healthy sexual life.

DISCLOSURE

The authors have nothing to disclose.

REFERENCES

1. World Health Organization. Sexual health throughout life: definition [Internet]. 2011. Available at: http://www.euro.who.int/en/health-topics/Life-stages/sexual-and-reproductive-health/news/news/2011/06/sexual-health-throughout-life/definition. Accessed January 31, 2020.
2. Stokes M, Kaur A. High-functioning autism and sexuality: a parental perspective. Autism 2005;9(3):266–89.
3. Dewinter J, De Graaf H, Beeger S. Sexual orientation, gender identity, and romantic relationships in adolescents and adults with autism spectrum disorder. J Autism Dev Disord 2017;47(9):2927–34.
4. Dewinter J, Vermeiren R, Vanwesenbeeck I, et al. Autism and normative sexual development: a narrative review. J Clin Nurs 2013;22:3467–83.
5. Schöttle D, Briken P, Tuescher O, et al. Sexuality in autism: hypersexual and paraphilic behaviour in women and men with high-functioning autism spectrum disorder. Dialogues Clin Neurosci 2017;19(4):381–93.
6. Lehan Mackin M, Loew N, Gonzalez A, et al. Parent perceptions of sexual education needs for their children with autism. J Pediatr Nurs 2016;31(6):608–18.
7. Stokes M, Newton N, Kaur A. Stalking, and social and romantic functioning among adolescents and adults with autism spectrum disorder. J Autism Dev Disord 2007;37(1):1969–86.
8. Allely CS, Creaby-Attwood A. Sexual offending and autism spectrum disorders. J Intellect Disabil Offending Behav 2016;7(1):35–51.
9. Wish JR, McCombs KF, Edmonson B. The socio-sexual knowledge, and attitudes test. Wood Dale (IL): Stoeling Co; 1980.

10. Chandra A, Mosher WD, Copen C. Sexual behavior, sexual attraction and sexual identity in the United States: data from the 2006-2008 national survey of family growth. Hyattsville (MD): United States: National Center for HIV/AIDS, Viral Hepatitis, STD, and TB Prevention; 2011.
11. Dewinter J, Vermeiren R, Vanwesenbeeck I, et al. Sexuality in adolescent boys with autism spectrum disorder: self-reported behaviours and attitudes. J Autism Dev Disord 2014;45(3):731–41.
12. Hellemans H, Colson K, Verbraeken C, et al. Sexual behavior in high-functioning male adolescents and young adults with autism spectrum disorder. J Autism Dev Disord 2007;37:260–9.
13. Van Bourgondien ME, Reichle NC, Palmer A. Sexual behavior in adults with autism. J Autism Dev Disord 1997;27(2):113–25.
14. Dewinter J, Vermeiren R, Vanwesenbeeck I, et al. Adolescent boys with autism spectrum disorder growing up: follow-up of self-reported sexual experience. Eur Child Adolesc Psychiatry 2016;25(9):969–78.
15. Byers ES, Nichols S, Voyer SD, et al. Sexual well-being of a community sample of high-functioning adults on the autism spectrum who have been in a romantic relationship. Autism 2013;17(4):418–33.
16. Robbins CL, Schick V, Reece M, et al. Prevalence, frequency, and associations of masturbation with partnered sexual behaviours among US adolescents. JAMA Pediatr 2011;165(12):1087–93.
17. Hénault I, Attwood T. The sexual profile of adults with Asperger's syndrome: the need for support and intervention. In: Hénault I, editor. Asperger's syndrome and sexuality: from adolescence to adulthood. London: Jessica Kingsley Publishers; 2006. p. 183–91.
18. Mehzabin P, Stokes MA. Self-assessed sexuality in young adults with high-functioning autism. Res Autism Spectr Disord 2011;5(1):614–21.
19. Bejerot S, Eriksson JM. Sexuality and gender role in autism spectrum disorder: a case control study. PLoS One 2014;9(1):e87961.
20. Dewinter J, Vermeiren R, Vanwesenbeeck I, et al. Parental awareness of sexual experience in adolescent boys with autism spectrum disorder. J Autism Dev Disord 2015;46(2):713–9.
21. May T, Pang KC, Williams K. Brief report: sexual attraction and relationships in adolescents with autism. J Autism Dev Disord 2017;47(6):1910–6.
22. Gilmour L, Schalomon PM, Smith V. Sexuality in a community based sample of adults with autism spectrum disorder. Res Autism Spectr Disord 2012;6(1):313–8.
23. Brown-Lavoie SM, Viecili MA, Weiss JA. Sexual knowledge and victimization in adults with autism spectrum disorders. J Autism Dev Disord 2014;44:2185–96.
24. Sevlever M, Roth ME, Gillis JM. Sexual abuse and offending in autism spectrum disorders. Sex Disabil 2013;31:189–200.
25. Weiss JA, Fardella MA. Victimization and perpetration experiences of adults with autism. Front Psychiatry 2018;25(9):203.
26. Stokes M, Newton N. Autism spectrum disorders and stalking. Autism 2004;8(3):337–9.
27. Chan J, John RM. Sexuality and sexual health in children and adolescents with autism. J Nurse Pract 2012;8(4):306–15.
28. Kellaher DC. Sexual behavior and autism spectrum disorders: an update and discussion. Curr Psychiatry Rep 2015;17(4):562.
29. Haracopos D, Pedersen L. Sexuality and autism: a national survey in Denmark. Copenhagen (Denmark): Center for Autism; 1992. Available at: http://www.autismuk.com/autisrn/sexuality-and-autism/sexuality-andautism-danish-report/.

30. Fernandes LC, Gillberg CI, Cederlund M, et al. Aspects of sexuality in adolescents and adults diagnosed with autism spectrum disorders in childhood. J Autism Dev Disord 2016;46(9):3155–65.
31. Chan LG, Saluja B. Sexual offending and improvement in autistic characteristics after acquired brain injury: a case report. Aust N Z J Psychiatry 2011;45(10): 902–3.
32. Griffin-Shelley E. Adolescent sex and love addicts. Westport (CT): Praeger Publishers; 1994.
33. Milton J, Duggan C, Latham A, et al. Case history of co-morbid Asperger's syndrome and paraphilic behavior. Med Sci Law 2002;42(3):237–44.
34. Loftin R, Westphal A, Sperry LA. Counterfeit deviance. In: Volkmar F, editor. Encyclopaedia of autism spectrum disorders. New York: Springer; 2018. p. 1–2.
35. Mahoney M. Asperger's syndrome and the criminal law: the special case of child pornography. 2009. Available at: https://www.harringtonmahoney.com/content/Publications/AspergersSyndromeandtheCriminalLawv26.pdf.   Accessed February 3, 2020.
36. Loftin R, Sperry L, Westphal A. Autism, the Internet and images of child exploitation. Washington, DC: National Center on Criminal Justice and Disability White Paper; 2015.
37. Loftin R, Westphal A, Sperry LA. Sexuality and problem behaviors. In: Volkmar F, editor. Encyclopedia of autism spectrum disorders. New York: Springer; 2018. https://doi.org/10.1007/978-1-4614-6435-8_102140-139.
38. Clark Mogavero M. Autism, sexual offending, and the criminal justice system. J Intellect Disabil Offending Behav 2016;7(3):116–26.
39. Allen D, Evans C, Hider A, et al. Offending behavior in adults with Asperger syndrome. J Autism Dev Disord 2008;38(4):748–58.
40. Mandell DS, Walrath CM, Manteuffel B, et al. The prevalence and correlates of abuse among children with autism served in comprehensive community-based mental health settings. Child Abuse Negl 2005;29:1359–72.
41. Pecora LA, Hancock GI, Mesibov GM, et al. Characterising the sexuality of autistic females. J Autism Dev Disord 2019;49(12):4834–46.
42. Ohlsson Gotby V, Lichtenstein P, Langström N, et al. Childhood neurodevelopmental disorders and risk of coercive sexual victimization in childhood and adolescence: a population-based prospective twin study. J Child Psychol Psychiatry 2018;59(9):957–65.
43. Braveheart: child sexual assault factsheet [Internet]. Australia: Bravehearts Foundation; 2019. Available at: https://bravehearts.org.au/wp-content/uploads/2019/10/WIP_Facts-and-stats_updated-Oct-2019.pdf. Accessed January 20, 2020.
44. Brown KR, Peña EV, Rankin S. Unwanted sexual contact: students with autism and other disabilities at greater risk. J Coll Stud Dev 2017;58:771–6.
45. Bush HH. Self-reported sexuality among women with and without autism spectrum disorder (ASD). Doctorate [dissertation]. Boston: University of Massachusetts; 2016.
46. Nichols S, Moravcik GM, Tetenbaum SP. Girls growing up on the autism spectrum. Philadelphia: Jessica Kingsley Publishers; 2008.
47. Paul A, Gallot C, Lelouche C, et al. Victimisation in a French population of children and youths with autism spectrum disorder: a case control study. Child Adolesc Psychiatry Ment Health 2018;12(48):1–23.
48. Gammicchia C, Johnson C. Autism: information for domestic violence and sexual assault counsellors. Bethesda (MD): Autism Society; 2014.

49. Attwood T. Girls and women who have Asperger's syndrome [Internet]. 2013. Available at: http://www.tonyattwood.com.au/index.php/about-aspergers/girls-and-women-who-have-aspergers. Accessed January 20, 2020.

50. Attwood T. Romantic relationships for young adults with Asperger syndrome and high-functioning autism [Internet]. 2009. Available at: https://iancommunity.org/cs/articles/relationships. Accessed January 20, 2020.

51. Cridland EK, Jones SC, Caputi P, et al. Being a girl in a boys' world: investigating the experiences of girls with autism spectrum disorders during adolescence. J Autism Dev Disord 2014;44:1261–74.

52. Roberts AL, Koenen KC, Lyall K, et al. Association of autistic traits in adulthood with childhood abuse, interpersonal victimization, and posttraumatic stress. Child Abuse Negl 2015;45:135–42.

53. Pecora LA, Hancock GI, Hooley M, et al. Gender identity, sexual orientation and adverse sexual experiences in autistic females. Mol Autism 2020.

54. Bargiela S, Steward R, Mandy W. The experiences of late-diagnosed women with autism spectrum conditions: an investigation of the female autism phenotype. J Autism Dev Disord 2016;46(10):3281–94.

55. George R, Stokes MA. A quantitative analysis of mental health among sexual and gender minorities in ASD. J Autism Dev Disord 2018;48(6):2052–63.

56. Collier KL, van Beusekom G, Bos HM, et al. Sexual orientation and gender identity/expression related peer victimization in adolescence: a systematic review of associated psychosocial and health outcomes. J Sex Res 2013;50(3–4):299–317.

57. Edelson MG. Sexual abuse of children with autism: factors that increase risk and interfere with recognition of abuse. Disabil Stud Q 2010;30(1). https://doi.org/10.18061/dsq.v30i1.1058.

58. Dennis M, Lockyer L, Lazenby AL. How high-functioning children with autism understand real and deceptive emotion. Autism 2000;4:370–81.

59. Bauminger N, Solomon M, Aviezer A, et al. Children with autism and their friends: a multidimensional study of friendship in high-functioning autism spectrum disorder. J Abnorm Child Psychol 2008;36(2):135–50.

60. George R, Stokes MA. Gender identity and sexual orientation in autism spectrum disorder. Autism 2017;22(8):970–82.

61. Byers SE, Nichols S, Voyer SD. Challenging stereotypes: sexual functioning of single adults with high functioning autism spectrum disorder. J Autism Dev Disord 2013;43(11):2617–27.

62. George R, Stokes MA. Sexual orientation in autism spectrum disorder. Autism Res 2018;11(1):133–41.

63. American Psychological Association. Guidelines for psychological practice with lesbian, gay, and bisexual clients. Am Psychol 2012;67(1):10–42.

64. Kelly G. A (nearly) complete glossary of gender identities for your next census [Internet]. 2016. Available at: https://www.telegraph.co.uk/men/the-filter/a-nearly-complete-glossary-of-gender-identities-for-your-next-ce/.   Accessed February 1, 2020.

65. American Psychological Association & National Association of School Psychologists. Resolution on gender and sexual orientation diversity in children and adolescents in schools [Internet]. 2015. Available at: http://www.apa.org/about/policy/orie ntation-diversity.aspx. Accessed January 21, 2020.

66. Rosario M, Schrimshaw EW. Theories and etiologies of sexual orientation. In: Tolman DL, Diamond LM, editors. APA handbook of sexuality and psychology – volume 1: person based approaches. Washington, DC: American Psychological Association; 2014. p. 555–96.

67. Adelson SL. Practice parameter on gay, lesbian, or bisexual sexual orientation, gender variance, and gender discordance in children and adolescents. J Am Acad Child Adolesc Psychiatry 2012;51(9):957–74.

68. Edwards-Leeper L, Spack NP. Psychological evaluation and medical treatment of transgender youth in an interdisciplinary "Gender Management Service" (GeMS) in a major pediatric center. J Homosex 2012;59:321–36.

69. Strang JF, Kenworthy L, Dominska A, et al. Increased gender variance in autism spectrum disorders and attention deficit hyperactivity disorder. Arch Sex Behav 2014;43(8):1525–33.

70. Janssen A, Huang H, Duncan C. Gender variance among youth with autism spectrum disorders: a retrospective chart review. Transgend Health 2016; 1(1):63–8.

71. Van der Miesen AIR, Hurley H, de Vries ALC. Gender dysphoria and autism spectrum disorder: a narrative review. Int Rev Psychiatry 2016;28(1):70–80.

72. American Psychiatric Association. Diagnostic and statistical manual of mental disorders. 5th edition. Arlington (VA): American Psychiatric Association; 2013.

73. Gallucci G, Hackerman F, Schmidt CW. Gender identity disorder in an adult male with Asperger's syndrome. Sex Disabil 2005;23(1):35–40.

74. Lemaire M, Thomazeau B, Bonnet-Brihault F. Gender identity disorder and autism spectrum disorder in a 23-year-old female. Arch Sex Behav 2014;43(2):395–8.

75. Parkinson J. Gender dysphoria in Asperger's syndrome: a caution. Australas Psychiatry 2014;22:84–5.

76. Jacobs LA, Rachlin K, Erickson-Schroth L, et al. Gender dysphoria and do-occurring autism spectrum disorders: review, case examples, and treatment considerations. LGBT Health 2014;1:277–82.

77. Landen M, Rasmussen P. Gender identity disorder in a girl with autism—a case report. Eur Child Adolesc Psychiatry 1997;6:170–3.

78. de Vries ALC, Noens ILJ, Cohen-Kettenis PT, et al. Autism spectrum disorders in gender dysphoric children and adolescents. J Autism Dev Disord 2010;40:930–6.

79. Centers for Disease Control and Prevention. Data & statistics on autism spectrum disorders. USA: U.S. Department of Health and Human Services; 2019. Available at: https://www.cdc.gov/ncbddd/autism/data.html. Accessed January 31, 2020.

80. Hartman CA, Luteijn E, Serra M, et al. Refinement of the Children's Social Behavior Questionnaire (CSBQ): an instrument that describes the diverse problems seen in milder forms of PDD. J Autism Dev Disord 2006;36:325–42.

81. van der Miesen AIR, de Vries ALC, Steensma TD, et al. Autistic symptoms in children and adolescents with gender dysphoria. J Autism Dev Disord 2018;48: 1537–48.

82. Baron-Cohen S, Wheelwright S, Skinner R, et al. The Autism-Spectrum Quotient (AQ): evidence from Asperger syndrome/high-functioning autism, males and females, scientists and mathematicians. J Autism Dev Disord 2001;31(1):5–17.

83. Pasterski V, Gilligan L, Curtis R. Traits of autism spectrum disorders in adults with gender dysphoria. Arch Sex Behav 2014;43:387–93.

84. Jones RM, Wheelwright S, Farrell K, et al. Brief report: female-to-male transsexual people and autistic traits. J Autism Dev Disord 2012;42(2):301–6.

85. Nobili A, Glazebrook C, Bouman WP, et al. Autistic traits in treatment-seeking transgender adults. J Autism Dev Disord 2018;48(12):3984–94.

86. Knickmeyer RC, Baron-Cohen S. Fetal testosterone and sex differences in typical social development in autism. J Child Neurol 2006;21(10):825–45.

87. Laugeson EA, Gantman A, Kapp SK, et al. A randomized controlled trial to improve social skills in young adults with autism spectrum disorder: the UCLA PEERS program. J Autism Dev Disord 2015;45(12):3978–89.

88. Planned Parenthood Federation of America. [Internet]. 2020. Available at: www.plannedparenthood.org. Accessed February 3, 2020.

89. Visser K, Greaves-Lord K, Tick NT, et al. A randomized controlled trial to examine the effects of the Tackling Teenage psychosexual training program for adolescents with autism spectrum disorder. J Child Psychol Psychiatry 2017;58(7):840–50.

90. Ballan MS, Freyer MB. Autism spectrum disorder, adolescence, and sexuality education: suggested interventions for mental health professionals. Sex Disabil 2017;35:261–73.

91. Scattone D, Wilczynski SM, Edwards RP, et al. Decreasing disruptive behaviors in children with autism using social stories. J Autism Dev Disord 2002;32(6):535–43.

92. Chen LP, Murad MH, Paras ML, et al. Sexual abuse and lifetime diagnosis of psychiatric disorders: systematic review and meta-analysis. Mayo Clin Proc 2010;85(7):618–29.

93. Morgan E. Preventing sexual victimization: an assertiveness training program for female adolescents. Doctorate [dissertation]. Kalamazoo (MI): Western Michigan University; 2018.

94. Mayer KH, Bradford JB, Makadon HJ, et al. Sexual and gender minority health: what we know and what needs to be done. Am J Public Health 2008;98(6):989–95.

95. Garthe RC, Hidalgo MA, Hereth J, et al. Prevalence and risk correlates of intimate partner violence among a multisite cohort of young transgender women. LGBT Health 2018;5(6):333–40.

Facial Expression Production and Recognition in Autism Spectrum Disorders
A Shifting Landscape

Connor Tom Keating, Jennifer Louise Cook, PhD (Neuroscience)*

KEYWORDS

- Autism spectrum disorder • Facial expression • Emotion recognition
- Emotion expression • Interaction • Alexithymia

KEY POINTS

- The social difficulties documented in autism spectrum disorder (ASD) may, in part, be a product of neurotypical-autistic differences (ie, differences in facial expressions).
- Neurotypical and autistic individuals typically exhibit expressive differences, with autistic individuals displaying less frequent expressions that are rated as lower in quality by non-autistic raters. It appears that alexithymia may contribute to these expressive differences.
- Autistic individuals have difficulties recognizing neurotypical facial expressions and vice versa.
- Task-related factors (eg, intensity of the emotional stimuli) and participant characteristics (eg, age, IQ, comorbid diagnoses and co-occurring alexithymia) may influence emotion recognition ability.
- Future research should investigate what specifically is different about the facial expressions produced by autistic and neurotypical individuals (eg, how dynamic aspects of expressions affect emotion recognition) and incorporate measures of alexithymia.

THE SHIFTING LANDSCAPE OF AUTISM RESEARCH AND ITS RELATIONSHIP WITH FACIAL EMOTION RESEARCH

Autism spectrum disorder (ASD) is a neurodevelopmental disorder, characterized by restricted and repetitive interests and difficulties with social communication and interaction.[1] Earlier research suggested that autistic people *lack* certain social abilities (including emotion recognition), and this absence of "social building blocks" led to social interaction difficulties in everyday situations (e.g., Refs.[2,3]). This view ignored the

This article originally appeared in *Child and Adolescent Psychiatric Clinics*, Volume 29, Issue 3, July 2020.
School of Psychology, University of Birmingham, Edgbaston, Birmingham B15 2TT, UK
* Corresponding author.
E-mail address: J.L.Cook@bham.ac.uk
Twitter: @ConnorTKeating (C.T.K.); @Jennifer_L_Cook (J.L.C.)

fact that social *interactions* are exactly that, an *interaction between individuals.* Autism research is now shifting towards an emphasis on the *differences* in certain abilities between autistic and neurotypical people. In the example of facial expression, when feeling sad, an autistic person might move their face into an expression that is not the downturned mouth expression that most neurotypical individuals would adopt. One consequence of this is that, because this expression is different from the norm, a neurotypical person might not recognize that the autistic person is feeling sad. Similarly, because the neurotypical person expresses their sadness in a different way from the autistic person, the autistic individual might not recognize the neurotypical individual's sadness. This "bidirectional" approach to evaluating social interactions leads to a consideration of both sides of the interaction.

Much of the research focusing on the bidirectional nature of social interactions in autism has emphasized body movement differences.[4,5] Arguably, the success and fluidity of an interaction depend on an accurate understanding and prediction of another's movement, facilitating the appropriate attribution of affective states (emotions) and intentions of the interaction partner.[6,7] Furthermore, we are better able to accurately infer emotional states/intentions, via nonverbal cues, when our interaction partner is someone who usually moves in a similar way to ourselves. Current literature indicates a high heterogeneity in the movement profiles of autistic individuals,[4] suggesting that autistic individuals move quite differently from both neurotypical and other autistic individuals.[4] Thus, the movement interpretation and resulting social interaction in autistic-autistic pairs may be no better than autistic-neurotypical pairs. Thus, what previously had been thought of as "social deficits" in autistic individuals may actually reflect a *mismatch* in movement profiles between autistic and neurotypical (or other autistic) individuals.

The mechanisms underpinning the difficulties in bidirectional emotion recognition depend on both emotion expression and emotion recognition. Typically, studies of emotion in autism have focused on the ability to perceive and label others' emotional expressions (ie, "emotion recognition"). However, recent evidence suggests that autistic and neurotypical individuals are less divergent in emotion recognition than in the active facial expression of emotion (ie, "emotion expression"), suggesting the latter is at least, if not more, important in the bidirectional misunderstanding of emotion.[8]

This review first asks whether there is evidence in support of the view that emotional expressions are different for autistic compared with neurotypical people. Second, the research assessing autistic individuals' emotion recognition (ie, recognition of neurotypical expressions) is reviewed. Finally, a small amount of research investigating neurotypical individuals' recognition of autistic expressions of emotion is discussed. Throughout, the authors identify factors that may be contributing to mixed findings in these literatures and highlight important areas for future research.

Facial Emotion Expression

Emotion expression in autism spectrum disorder

Key components to consider when examining whether autistic individuals exhibit differences in emotional expression include the frequency and duration of the expressions and the intensity of the emotional expressions (expressiveness). Meta-analytic, and numerous empirical, studies suggest that during naturalistic social interactions autistic children typically display facial expressions less often and for a shorter duration compared with non-autistic children.[9–12] In terms of expressiveness, autistic and neurotypical individuals exhibit comparable intensities of expression.[12] Several studies report no differences in facial expressiveness between autistic and neurotypical individuals during automatic imitation (as measured by motion tracking),[13] while participants view emotional stimuli (eg, images, videos),[14–16] and when mimicking emotional facial expressions[17,18] (as measured by facial electromyography). These latter findings suggest that differences in emotion production are more likely due to atypical spontaneous productions as opposed to a physical inability to produce appropriate expressions.[19] Autistic individuals may execute expressions that are visually different (ie, using different parts of their face), less accurate (ie, socially incongruous), or lower in quality (as rated by typical observers/experimenters) rather than simply lower intensity.

In line with this interpretation, numerous studies report that autistic individuals produce spontaneous expressions that are perceived as lower in *quality,* and rated as odd, stilted, or mechanical by non-autistic observers and experimenters.[10,19–21] Research concerning mimicry of facial expressions has demonstrated that, compared with non-autistic children, those with ASD mimic facial expressions *less accurately* (ie, with lower congruency).[17,22] Therefore, it appears that autistic individuals have the physical capacity to mimic facial expressions; however, when they do, the expressions are of lower quality.[a] In line with this, recent meta-analytic data suggest that facial expressions of autistic individuals are less accurate and are lower in quality relative to controls.[12] Overall, it appears that autistic individuals display facial expressions less frequently and for a shorter duration, and when they do so they are less accurate and lower in quality as rated by non-autistic observers.

Although there is evidence that autistic and neurotypical individuals exhibit expressive differences, research has not yet identified *what* specifically is different about these facial expressions. Facial expressions can be quantified in several ways. One could look at the final arrangement of facial features and ask whether there are *spatial* differences between expressions produced by autistic and non-autistic individuals (eg, one group might open their mouth further when smiling to express happiness). One can also ask whether there are *kinematic* differences between groups (eg, when expressing happiness, one group might break into a smile more quickly). Although autistic and neurotypical facial expressions could, in principle, differ in terms of spatial or kinematic features, to the best of the authors' knowledge, studies have not specifically aimed to assess the contributions of these two factors. Future research to characterize the spatial and kinematic expressive differences between ASD and comparison groups could lead to a better understanding of autistic facial emotional expression. Such research results could be used to better train caregivers and clinicians to interpret autistic facial expressions, thus facilitating more successful social interactions.

Alexithymia and emotion expression

Alexithymia is a subclinical condition characterized by difficulties identifying, expressing, and differentiating emotions.[23] Recent evidence suggests that, across both neurotypical and autistic populations, alexithymia may be implicated in the production of atypical facial expressions. Approximately 50% of the autistic population experiences co-occurring alexithymia[24] in comparison to just 14% of the typical population.[25] The "alexithymia hypothesis" postulates that difficulties in emotion processing in ASD are caused by co-occurring alexithymia, rather than ASD itself.[26] This hypothesis builds on the observation that the systems responsible for the experience of a particular

---

[a] Note that, given that non-imitative autistic facial expressions tend to be rated low in quality/accuracy, these results cannot be taken as evidence of atypical *imitation* mechanisms. It is more likely that they reflect differences in emotional expression.

emotion contribute to the recognition of the same emotion in others.[27–29] The alexithymia hypothesis highlights that alexithymic individuals, by definition, exhibit differences in experiencing their own emotions (eg, difficulties with labeling their emotions), and this has a "knock-on effect" on the ability to recognize others' emotions.

Alexithymia has been associated with reduced quantity of facial expressions produced by both autistic and neurotypical individuals. A recent study, using iMotion's facial expression analysis technology[30] to estimate the extent to which an emotion is being expressed at any given time, examined the contributions of several variables on emotion expression in autistic and non-autistic children.[31] This study identified that alexithymia (as measured by the Children's Alexithymia Measure[32]), and not intelligence quotient (IQ, sex, or ASD traits, predicted the between-subject variance in the facial expressions produced by child participants.[31] Despite some mixed findings, these results are consistent with studies investigating populations without ASD.[33–36] For example, increased alexithymia is associated with diminished production of facial expressions by patients during therapeutic interaction[33] and production of less salient facial expressions in undergraduate students as evaluated by trained raters.[34] Overall, it appears that alexithymia is implicated in the production of facial expressions across multiple populations. Future studies investigating facial emotion expression in autism must account for the potential co-occurrence of alexithymia.

Facial Emotion Recognition

Recognition of others' emotions in autism spectrum disorder
Emotion recognition has been a topic of interest in autism research for more than 30 years, with studies generally documenting difficulties in the autistic population. Indeed, recent research indicates that ASD-related facial expression recognition[b] difficulties are present cross-culturally, illustrating that emotion recognition difficulties are widespread in the autistic population.[37] In addition, recent meta-analytic evidence finds robust emotion recognition difficulties in ASD,[38,39] with the latter incorporating 43 studies (41 of which used static stimuli with posed expressions, and 40 of which used forced-choice tasks) with more than 1500 participants. Nevertheless, this literature is rife with conflicting findings,[40–45] with some studies reporting profound difficulties and others reporting no differences between autistic and neurotypical participants (see Refs.[38,39,46] for reviews). Several factors may account for variation in findings across ASD facial emotion recognition studies.

Task-related factors
Intensity of emotional expressions Differences in the intensity of facial expression stimuli may influence facial expression recognition ability[47–49] and hence may contribute to inconsistencies in research findings. Most studies that have failed to find emotion recognition difficulties in ASD (eg, Refs.[40–45]) have used 100% intensity, or "full-blown" emotional expressions. Therefore, it is possible that the tasks used were not sufficiently sensitive to detect ASD-comparison group differences and were confounded by ceiling effects. Relatively few studies have directly compared the facial expression recognition ability of autistic and neurotypical individuals across different intensity levels. The findings from studies that have done so are mixed, with conflicting evidence suggesting difficulties recognizing low-, but not high-intensity expressions,[47–49] and difficulties with medium-, but not low-/high-intensity expressions.[50] Some studies suggest no effect of expression intensity on facial expression

---

[b] In the literature, the terms "facial affect recognition" and "facial emotion recognition" are also used. In this review, "facial expression recognition" will be used to refer to all of these terms.

recognition in ASD.[51–53] Importantly, many of the studies that suggest differential impairment as a function of expression intensity have used small samples (often <20 in the ASD group). Two more recent studies with larger sample sizes (N = 95 and N = 127, respectively) indicate that young autistic individuals (aged 6–14 and 6–16, respectively) were less accurate than young neurotypical individuals at labeling basic (happy, surprise, angry, sad, fear, disgust) emotional expressions across all intensity levels,[51,54] even though both neurotypical and autistic individuals had better facial expression recognition as the intensity of the expressions increased. Future studies should investigate the emotion recognition ability of autistic adults across various intensity levels.

Static versus dynamic stimuli Two broad types of stimuli are commonly used to investigate facial expression recognition: static and dynamic. Because spontaneous facial expressions are inherently dynamic, dynamic depictions are presumed to have higher ecological validity.[39,55] Moreover, given that studies using dynamic tasks are greatly underrepresented in meta-analyses (about 21% of studies included in Uljarevic and Hamilton[39] and just 0%–5% in Lozier and colleagues[38]), greater inclusion of dynamic stimuli in future research is necessary.[55] Although this assertion is true, the authors believe that there is also great utility in using *both* static and dynamic stimuli to assess emotion recognition. Incorporating both types of tasks allows one to distinguish whether autistic individuals have difficulties with processing static (ie, the configuration of facial features relative to each other) or dynamic (ie, speed of movement of features, or temporal order of face movements) features of facial expressions. Krumhuber and colleagues[55] point out that the benefits of viewing dynamic (as oppose to static) stimuli are most apparent when subtle expressions are used. Consequently, it appears that when expressions are less intense, there is greater reliance on the dynamic features of facial expressions. More research, however, is necessary to understand the extent to which, and under what conditions (eg, for subtle emotions), *autistic* individuals specifically rely on dynamic versus static information in facial emotion recognition tasks.

The few studies that have examined the processing of dynamic facial information indicate autistic-neurotypical differences. One study identified that autistic individuals tended to rate slow moving morphs as more "natural looking" than neurotypicals.[56] Another study used a professional actress to slowly portray emotional (joy, surprise, sadness, and disgust) and non-emotional (pronunciation of 3 vowels A, O, I, and tongue protrusion) expressions. The velocity of the videos was then artificially manipulated to give 3 conditions: "normal condition" (accelerated), "slow condition" (the filmed version), and "very slow" (deaccelerated).[57] Although, in the primary analyses, the autistic children exhibited lower facial expression recognition than verbal age-matched and nonverbal age-matched controls for both the emotional and the non-emotional stimuli, they had even lower accuracy with the emotional stimuli.[57] In post-hoc analyses, the investigators found that the autistic group had better emotional facial expression recognition in the slow relative to the normal speed condition.[57] Indeed, further post hoc analyses demonstrated that children with moderate to severe autism (ie, with Childhood Autism Rating Scale[58] scores ≥35 in this study) had better performance when the expressions were displayed slowly and/or very slowly.[57] As a whole, the investigators comment that each autistic child will have their own pattern of "perceptual and cognitive reactivity to the speed of facial motion," with slow presentations generally being most easily recognized.[57] More research, which formally uses a control group in their statistical comparisons, is necessary to elucidate whether enhancements in facial expression recognition for slowed facial stimuli are ASD-specific.

In sum, although there is a paucity of research in this area, a handful of studies suggest differences in processing dynamic aspects of facial expressions in autism.

Findings from behavioral investigations of dynamic expression processing in autism resonate well with those from neurophysiological studies. Although there is some inconsistency,[59] and caution is advised, this literature indicates that, relative to neurotypicals, autistic individuals display slowed processing of static face images as indexed by N170 latency.[60–64] It is possible there is a link between slowed neural processing of facial information in ASD, enhanced recognition of slow-moving faces,[57] and the perception that slow-moving faces are more natural looking.[56] Future studies that combine behavioral and neurophysiological investigations are necessary.

In conclusion, it appears that differences in emotion recognition are evident between autistic and neurotypical individuals for both static and dynamic stimuli, and hence, it is unlikely that use of differing stimuli types contributes to the mixed findings. Importantly, however, it appears that dynamic stimuli confer the greatest benefit when expressions are low intensity, suggesting a reliance on dynamic information when viewing subtle expressions. The evidence from neurophysiological studies and studies using dynamic tasks suggests that autistic individuals may exhibit slowed processing of facial information. More research using dynamic stimuli, however, is necessary to confirm whether the kinematic properties of face stimuli specifically influence facial expression recognition ability.

Participant characteristics

Age and intelligence quotient In addition to task demands, participant characteristics (eg, age and IQ) may influence the presence and magnitude of emotion recognition differences in ASD.[46] Although emotion recognition improves throughout life for neurotypicals,[65] studies suggest that this may not be true for autistic individuals.[65] In accordance, a recent meta-analysis divided the existing studies that have investigated emotion recognition into those that assessed pediatric (younger than 18 years) and those that assessed adult autistic participants.[38] In both groups, there were differences in emotion recognition relative to neurotypical participants (who had been age-matched in 32 of the 41 studies used for these age-based analyses); however, differences were greater in the adult group than in the pediatric group.[38] Furthermore, when these researchers modeled the mean participant age in each study as a predictor in a linear regression, age was a significant predictor of emotion recognition accuracy in the regression model.[38] Such results suggest a widening gap in emotion recognition ability between neurotypical and autistic individuals as they grow older.

IQ is also implicated in the emotion recognition ability of both autistic and neurotypical individuals. Individuals with a higher IQ tend to have better emotion recognition.[66,67] High intelligence may buffer against emotion recognition difficulties[68] (**Fig. 1**).

Overall, it appears that although neurotypicals improve in their emotion recognition with age, this is not the case for autistic individuals, thus resulting in greater group differences in adulthood. The interaction between age and IQ is important to consider, especially because it seems that autistic and neurotypical individuals proceed along different developmental trajectories, and so compensatory mechanisms (e.g., IQ) may be more important at later developmental stages when there is a greater disparity in emotion recognition.[38]

Comorbidities Comorbid conditions may influence the presence and extent of differences in emotion recognition between autistic and neurotypical individuals. For instance, Sinzig and colleagues[69] showed that individuals with ASD and comorbid attention deficit hyperactivity disorder (ADHD) symptoms showed greater differences,

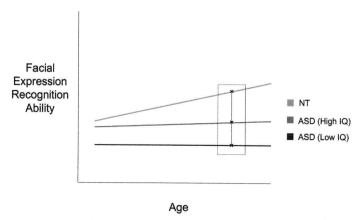

Fig. 1. The developmental trajectory of facial expression recognition ability between neuro-typical (*green*), high IQ autistic (*orange*), and low IQ autistic (*purple*) individuals. Note that the purple and orange lines are flat as evidence suggests no age effect for autistic individuals; however, the evidence is limited. The crosses and line represent that participants must be age- and IQ-matched. If participants are not matched on these factors, then the impact of ASD (above and beyond that of age and IQ) on facial expression recognition cannot be suitably examined. NT, neurotypical.

relative to neurotypicals, in facial expression recognition than those with only ASD.[69] Similarly, subclinical ADHD traits, such as attentional distractibility, are associated with facial expression recognition atypicalities in autistic participants.[70] Thus, ADHD-related traits may increase the likelihood of experiencing difficulties with facial expression recognition. High comorbidity between ASD and ADHD (29%[71]) may result in apparent expression recognition differences between autistic and neurotypical populations, which more accurately reflect the presence or absence of ADHD (not ASD) -related traits.

A similar argument has been forwarded for traits related to mood disorders. For instance, response biases toward negative emotions have been documented in mood-related disorders, such as anxiety and depression,[72,73] which are known to co-occur with ASD.[74] Negative emotion response biases have been identified when autistic individuals complete forced choice labeling tasks[51] (which are commonly used in the emotion recognition literature). Hence, Evers and colleagues[51] emphasize the impact of response biases and suggest that they may account for the inconsistent results between studies. Mood disorder–related traits may therefore comprise a further characteristic that biases individuals toward experiencing difficulties with facial expression recognition. Further research is necessary to assess the extent to which mood disorder–related traits contribute to expression recognition in autism. Response biases tend to be amplified with low-intensity and ambiguous stimuli.[54,75] Future studies might use low-intensity/ambiguous expressions to gain an estimate of bias, which can then be taken into account when comparing differences in facial expression recognition between groups.[54]

Co-occurring alexithymia may contribute to emotion recognition difficulties in individuals with ASD. Indeed, alexithymia is associated with emotion recognition difficulties in neurotypical populations (see Grynberg and colleagues[76] for a review), even after controlling for depression and anxiety scores.[77] Furthermore, because rates of alexithymia are higher in autistic than in non-autistic populations,[23,24] alexithymia may contribute to apparent emotion recognition differences between these populations. In line with this, research has demonstrated that, after controlling for alexithymia, attentional biases away from the eyes,[78] and emotion recognition difficulties[79] are no longer associated with ASD. Moreover, Cook and colleagues[79] found that possessing alexithymic traits, and not ASD traits, predicted poorer emotion recognition. Therefore, it appears that emotion recognition difficulties typically attributed to autism may be associated with co-occurring alexithymia rather than ASD itself.

Neurotypical Recognition of Autistic Expressions

Although there are several studies in which neurotypical raters/experimenters/research assistants have rated the quality, intensity, or accuracy of autistic facial emotional expressions (for example, Refs.[19–21]) very few studies have specifically aimed to evaluate whether neurotypical individuals have difficulty recognizing autistic facial expressions.[5,19,21,80] Most of those who have done so report difficulties for neurotypicals in recognizing autistic expressions.[5,21,80] For instance, Brewer and colleagues[5] asked autistic and neurotypical participants to match facial expressions that had been posed by autistic and neurotypical individuals with 1 of 6 prompted emotions. Interestingly, a "same-group" advantage was identified for the neurotypical but not the autistic group.[5] That is, neurotypical participants more accurately matched expressions produced by other neurotypical individuals, but performed more poorly when it came to recognizing the expressions of autistic individuals. Such findings are paralleled in the work of Edey and colleagues,[4] which investigated arm movements. In this experiment, autistic and neurotypical participants used magnetic levers to animate shapes such that they depicted mental state interactions (eg, fighting, following). Edey and colleagues[4] observed that neurotypical individuals accurately recognized the mental states depicted in animations produced by other neurotypical participants, but not by autistic participants. Therefore, it appears that in a similar way to how autistic individuals may have difficulties inferring others' emotion,[38,39,46] neurotypicals may also find it difficult to read and interpret autistic facial expressions and bodily movements.

SUMMARY AND FUTURE DIRECTIONS

Autism research is turning away from a focus on a lack of emotion recognition skills in autistic individuals and orienting toward the view that emotion processing depends on common representations of emotions between interaction partners. In line with this, the authors asked the following three key questions.

1. Does evidence support the idea that emotional expressions are different for autistic compared with neurotypical people?
   The studies reviewed provide evidence that there are broad differences between autistic and neurotypical individuals. The extant literature indicates that, in social situations, autistic individuals execute facial expressions less frequently,[12] and neurotypical individuals rate autistic expressions as lower in quality compared with neurotypical expressions.[12] Importantly, recent research suggests that alexithymia is implicated in the production of facial expressions; however, more research is necessary to clarify the extent of this involvement. Moreover, the way in which autistic expressions differ from neurotypical expressions is currently unclear. Future research should aim to elucidate *what* specifically is different about facial expressions produced by autistic and neurotypical individuals by assessing the spatial and kinematic properties of these expressions.

2. To what extent can autistic individuals recognize neurotypical emotional expressions?

   The evidence also indicates atypicalities. However, this is a very mixed literature: In some studies, autistic individuals display emotion recognition performance that does not differ from that of neurotypical individuals, whereas other studies report considerable differences.[46] Both task requirements (eg, differences in the intensity of emotional expressions) and individual differences (eg, age, IQ, comorbidities, alexithymia, and so forth) may influence the presence and severity of emotion recognition difficulties. Comorbidities, such as depression and alexithymia, are particularly important to consider because an autistic individual who also experiences one of these conditions is likely to exhibit facial emotion recognition difficulties, although such difficulties are more likely associated with the comorbid condition than with autism per se. To bring clarity to this research field, it is important that future research controls for comorbidities like alexithymia[81] and makes use of *dynamic* tasks, which facilitate the investigation of temporal and kinematic aspects involved in facial expression recognition. Such research will elucidate whether expression recognition differences are (a) present in individuals that are autistic and have no comorbidities, and (b) due to differences in the processing of spatial, temporal, or kinematic information. Future research has the power to, for example, clarify whether autistic individuals exhibit slowed processing of facial stimuli. Results may have significant implications: for example, if studies indicate slowed processing of emotional information in ASD, interventions could be designed to train caregivers and clinicians to move their faces more slowly when conveying emotional messages. Crucially, this could scaffold interpersonal abilities and elevate social competency, which could lead to greater social participation and lower social isolation.[82]

3. To what extent can neurotypical individuals recognize autistic emotional expressions?

   The evidence indicates that neurotypical individuals may have difficulties reading and interpreting autistic facial expressions and bodily movements. However, to date, there are very few studies addressing neurotypical recognition of autistic emotions. Further research is necessary to advance the understanding of the magnitude and consequences of these neurotypical-autistic emotion recognition difficulties.

Overall, this review suggests that, in the laboratory, there are bidirectional difficulties between autistic and neurotypical individuals in reading each other's facial expressions (**Fig. 2**).[5] Consequently, it may be the case that autistic and neurotypical faces are essentially "speaking a different language" with respect to conveying emotions. If this is indeed the case, there are several corresponding practical implications. For instance, caregivers and clinicians could be trained to "read the language" of autistic facial expressions, leading to a reduction in bidirectional sociocommunicative difficulties. Furthermore, as Edey and colleagues[4] argue, these bidirectional sociocommunicative difficulties have important implications for the clinical diagnosis of autism. Thus far, ASD has been diagnosed following observational behavioral assessments of social ability by a qualified clinician. However, it is possible that individuals may be evaluated, by non-autistic clinicians, as lacking in expression when, in reality, they have an incompatible movement profile with the assessor. To give an example, a nonverbal individual may be attempting to communicate via their facial expressions that they are happy but, if the expression is one that the clinician is unfamiliar with

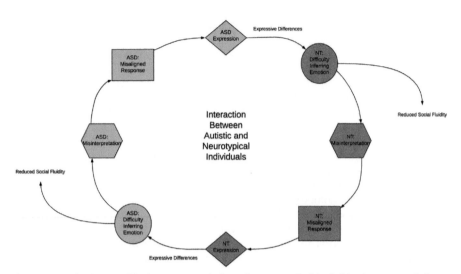

Fig. 2. How the interaction between autistic and neurotypical individuals may result in social difficulties.

and would not use in his/her own behavioral repertoire, he or she may conclude that the individual is not exhibiting the correct emotion. Thus, a *different* style of emotional expression is falsely interpreted as a *lack* of emotional expression. In conclusion, it appears that the view of emotion recognition in ASD is shifting away from the idea of "deficit" toward one of "difference" resulting from neurotypical-autistic *interactions*.

DISCLOSURE

The authors have nothing to disclose. This project was supported by the Medical Research Council (MRC, United Kingdom) MR/R015813/1 and the European Union's Horizon 2020 Research and Innovation Programme under ERC-2017-STG Grant Agreement No 757583.

REFERENCES

1. American Psychiatric Association. Diagnostic and statistical manual of mental disorders. 5th edition (DSM-5). Arlington, VA: American Psychiatric Association; 2013.
2. Schultz RT, Grelotti DJ, Klin A, et al. The role of the fusiform face area in social cognition: implications for the pathobiology of autism. Philos Trans R Soc B Biol Sci 2003;358(1430):415–27.
3. Hobson RP. The autistic child's appraisal of expressions of emotion. J Child Psychol Psychiatry 1986;27(3):321–42.
4. Edey R, Cook J, Brewer R, et al. Interaction takes two: typical adults exhibit mindblindness towards those with autism spectrum disorder. J Abnorm Psychol 2016; 125(7):879–85.
5. Brewer R, Biotti F, Catmur C, et al. Can neurotypical individuals read autistic facial expressions? Atypical production of emotional facial expressions in autism spectrum disorders. Autism Res 2016;9(2):262–71.

6. Halberstadt AG, Denham SA, Dunsmore JC. Affective social competence. Soc Dev 2001;10(1):79–119.

7. Behrends A, Müller S, Dziobek I. Moving in and out of synchrony: a concept for a new intervention fostering empathy through interactional movement and dance. Arts Psychother 2012;39(2):107–16.

8. Grossman RB, Tager-Flusberg H. Quality matters! Differences between expressive and receptive non-verbal communication skills in adolescents with ASD. Res Autism Spectr Disord 2012;6(3):1150–5.

9. Czapinski P, Bryson SE. Reduced facial muscle movements in autism: evidence for dysfunction in the neuromuscular pathway? Brain Cogn 2003;51(2):177–9.

10. Loveland KA, Tunali-Kotoski B, Pearson DA, et al. Imitation and expression of facial affect in autism. Dev Psychopathol 1994;6(3):433–44.

11. Kasari C, Sigman M, Mundy P, et al. Affective sharing in the context of joint attention interactions of normal, autistic, and mentally retarded children. J Autism Dev Disord 1990;20(1):87–100.

12. Trevisan DA, Hoskyn M, Birmingham E. Facial expression production in autism: a meta-analysis. Autism Res 2018;11(12):1586–601.

13. Press C, Richardson D, Bird G. Intact imitation of emotional facial actions in autism spectrum conditions. Neuropsychologia 2010;48(11):3291–7.

14. Deschamps PKH, Coppes L, Kenemans JL, et al. Electromyographic responses to emotional facial expressions in 6–7 year olds with autism spectrum disorders. J Autism Dev Disord 2013;45(2):354–62.

15. Magnée MJCM, De Gelder B, Van Engeland H, et al. Facial electromyographic responses to emotional information from faces and voices in individuals with pervasive developmental disorder. J Child Psychol Psychiatry 2007;48(11):1122–30.

16. Rozga A, King TZ, Vuduc RW, et al. Undifferentiated facial electromyography responses to dynamic, audio-visual emotion displays in individuals with autism spectrum disorders. Dev Sci 2013;16(4):499–514.

17. McIntosh DN, Reichmann-Decker A, Winkielman P, et al. When the social mirror breaks: deficits in automatic, but not voluntary, mimicry of emotional facial expressions in autism. Dev Sci 2006;9(3):295–302.

18. Oberman LM, Winkielman P, Ramachandran VS. Slow echo: facial EMG evidence for the delay of spontaneous, but not voluntary, emotional mimicry in children with autism spectrum disorders. Dev Sci 2009;12(4):510–20.

19. Faso DJ, Sasson NJ, Pinkham AE. Evaluating posed and evoked facial expressions of emotion from adults with autism spectrum disorder. J Autism Dev Disord 2014;45(1):75–89.

20. Grossman RB, Edelson LR, Tager-Flusberg H. Emotional facial and vocal expressions during story retelling by children and adolescents with high-functioning autism. J Speech Lang Hear Res 2013;56(3):1035–44.

21. Macdonald H, Rutter M, Howlin P, et al. Recognition and expression of emotional cues by autistic and normal adults. J Child Psychol Psychiatry 1989;30(6):865–77.

22. Yoshimura S, Sato W, Uono S, et al. Impaired overt facial mimicry in response to dynamic facial expressions in high-functioning autism spectrum disorders. J Autism Dev Disord 2015;45(5):1318–28.

23. Nemiah JC, Freyberger H, Sifneos PE. Alexithymia: a view of the psychosomatic process. Modern Trends in Psychosomatic Medicine 1976;3:430–9.

24. Berthoz S, Hill EL. The validity of using self-reports to assess emotion regulation abilities in adults with autism spectrum disorder. Eur Psychiatry 2005;20(3): 291–8.

25. Salminen JK, Saarijärvi S, Äärelä E, et al. Prevalence of alexithymia and its association with sociodemographic variables in the general population of Finland. J Psychosom Res 1999;46(1):75–82.

26. Bird G, Cook R. Mixed emotions: the contribution of alexithymia to the emotional symptoms of autism. Transl Psychiatry 2013;3(7):e285–8.

27. Adolphs R, Tranel D, Damasio H, et al. Impaired recognition of emotion in facial expressions following bilateral damage to the human amygdala. Neurocase 1997;3(4):267a–274.

28. Calder AJ, Lawrence AD, Young AW. Neuropsychology of fear and loathing. Nat Rev Neurosci 2001;2(5):352–63.

29. Calder AJ, Young AW. Understanding the recognition of facial identity and facial expression. Nat Rev Neurosci 2005;6(8):641–51.

30. iMotions biometric research platform 5.7, iMotion A/S, Copenhagen, Denmark. 2016. Available at: https://help.imotions.com/hc/en-us/articles/208460695-How-to-Cite-iMotions. Accessed November 15, 2019.

31. Trevisan DA, Bowering M, Birmingham E. Alexithymia, but not autism spectrum disorder, may be related to the production of emotional facial expressions. Mol Autism 2016;7:46.

32. Way IF, Applegate B, Cai X, et al. Children's alexithymia measure (CAM): a new instrument for screening difficulties with emotional expression. J Child Adolesc Trauma 2011;4(3):258.

33. Rasting M, Brosig B, Beutel ME. Alexithymic characteristics and patient-therapist interaction: a video analysis of facial affect display. Psychopathology 2005;38(3): 105–11.

34. Wagner H, Lee V. Alexithymia and individual differences in emotional expression. J Res Pers 2008;42(1):83–95.

35. Berenbaum H, Irvin S. Alexithymia, anger, and interpersonal behaviour. Psychother Psychosom 1996;65(4):203–8.

36. McDonald PW, Prkachin K. The expression and perception of facial emotion in alexithymia: a pilot study. Psychosom Med 1990;52(2):199–210.

37. Fridenson-Hayo S, Berggren S, Lassalle A, et al. Basic and complex emotion recognition in children with autism: cross-cultural findings. Mol Autism 2016; 7(1):1–11.

38. Lozier LM, Vanmeter JW, Marsh AA. Impairments in facial affect recognition associated with autism spectrum disorders: a meta-analysis. Dev Psychopathol 2014; 26(4):933–45.

39. Uljarevic M, Hamilton A. Recognition of emotions in autism: a formal meta-analysis. J Autism Dev Disord 2013;43(7):1517–26.

40. Baron-Cohen S, Jolliffe T, Mortimore C, et al. Another advanced test of theory of mind: evidence from very high functioning adults with autism or Asperger syndrome. J Child Pscyhol Psychiatry 1997;38:813–22.

41. Castelli F. Understanding emotions from standardized facial expressions in autism and normal development. Autism 2005;9(4):428–49.

42. Jones CRG, Pickles A, Falcaro M, et al. A multimodal approach to emotion recognition ability in autism spectrum disorders. J Child Psychol Psychiatry 2011;52(3): 275–85.

43. Da Fonseca D, Santos A, Bastard-Rosset D, et al. Can children with autistic spectrum disorders extract emotions out of contextual cues? Res Autism Spectr Disord 2009;3(1):50–6.
44. Neumann D, Spezio ML, Piven J, et al. Looking you in the mouth: abnormal gaze in autism resulting from impaired top-down modulation of visual attention. Soc Cogn Affect Neurosci 2006;1(3):194–202.
45. Spezio ML, Adolphs R, Hurley RSE, et al. Abnormal use of facial information in high-functioning autism. J Autism Dev Disord 2007;37(5):929–39.
46. Harms MB, Martin A, Wallace GL. Facial emotion recognition in autism spectrum disorders: a review of behavioral and neuroimaging studies. Neuropsychol Rev 2010;20(3):290–322.
47. Wong N, Beidel DC, Sarver DE, et al. Facial emotion recognition in children with high functioning autism and children with social phobia. Child Psychiatry Hum Dev 2012;43(5):775–94.
48. Ogai M, Matsumoto H, Suzuki K, et al. fMRI study of recognition of facial expressions in high-functioning autistic patients. Neuroreport 2003;14(4):559–63.
49. Wallace GL, Case LK, Harms MB, et al. Diminished sensitivity to sad facial expressions in high functioning autism spectrum disorders is associated with symptomatology and adaptive functioning. J Autism Dev Disord 2011;41(11):1475–86.
50. Doi H, Fujisawa TX, Kanai C, et al. Recognition of facial expressions and prosodic cues with graded emotional intensities in adults with asperger syndrome. J Autism Dev Disord 2013;43(9):2099–113.
51. Evers K, Steyaert J, Noens I, et al. Reduced recognition of dynamic facial emotional expressions and emotion-specific response bias in children with an autism spectrum disorder. J Autism Dev Disord 2015;45(6):1774–84.
52. Kessels RPC, Spee P, Hendriks AW. Perception of dynamic facial emotional expressions in adolescents with autism spectrum disorders (ASD). Transl Neurosci 2010;1(3):228–32.
53. Ketelaars MP, In'T Velt A, Mol A, et al. Emotion recognition and alexithymia in high functioning females with autism spectrum disorder. Res Autism Spectr Disord 2016;21:51–60.
54. Griffiths S, Jarrold C, Penton-Voak IS, et al. Impaired recognition of basic emotions from facial expressions in young people with autism spectrum disorder: assessing the importance of expression intensity. J Autism Dev Disord 2019;49(7):2768–78.
55. Krumhuber EG, Kappas A, Manstead ASR. Effects of dynamic aspects of facial expressions: a review. Emot Rev 2013;5(1):41–6.
56. Sato W, Uono S, Toichi M. Atypical recognition of dynamic changes in facial expressions in autism spectrum disorders. Res Autism Spectr Disord 2013;7(7):906–12.
57. Tardif C, Lainé F, Rodriguez M, et al. Slowing down presentation of facial movements and vocal sounds enhances facial expression recognition and induces facial-vocal imitation in children with autism. J Autism Dev Disord 2008;41:1469–84.
58. Schopler E, Reichler RJ, de Vellis RF, et al. Toward objective classification of childhood autism: Childhood Autism Rating Scale (CARS). J Autism Dev Disord 1980;10:91–103.
59. Webb SJ, Jones EJH, Merkle K, et al. Response to familiar faces, newly familiar faces, and novel faces as assessed by ERPs is intact in adults with autism spectrum disorders. Int J Psychophysiol 2010;77(2):106–17.

60. Hileman CM, Henderson H, Mundy P, et al. Developmental and individual differences on the P1 and N170 ERP components in children with and without autism. Dev Neuropsychol 2011;36(2):214–36.
61. McPartland J, Dawson G, Webb SJ, et al. Event-related brain potentials reveal anomalies in temporal processing of faces in autism spectrum disorder. J Child Psychol Psychiatry 2004;45(7):1235–45.
62. O'Connor K, Hamm JP, Kirk IJ. The neurophysiological correlates of face processing in adults and children with Asperger's syndrome. Brain Cogn 2005; 59(1):82–95.
63. O'Connor K, Hamm JP, Kirk IJ. Neurophysiological responses to face, facial regions and objects in adults with Asperger's syndrome: an ERP investigation. Int J Psychophysiol 2007;63(3):283–93.
64. Webb SJ, Dawson G, Bernier R, et al. ERP evidence of atypical face processing in young children with autism. J Autism Dev Disord 2006;36(7):881–90.
65. Rump KM, Giovannelli JL, Minshew NJ, et al. The development of emotion recognition in individuals with autism. Child Dev 2009;80(5):1434–47.
66. Dyck MJ, Piek JP, Hay D, et al. Are abilities abnormally interdependent in children with autism? J Clin Child Adolesc Psychol 2006;35:20–33.
67. Wright B, Clarke N, Jordan J, et al. Emotion recognition in faces and the use of visual context in young people with high-functioning autism spectrum disorders. Autism 2008;12(6):607–26.
68. Rutherford MD, Troje NF. IQ predicts biological motion perception in autism spectrum disorders. J Autism Dev Disord 2012;42(4):557–65.
69. Sinzig J, Morsch D, Lehmkuhl G. Do hyperactivity, impulsivity and inattention have an impact on the ability of facial affect recognition in children with autism and ADHD? Eur Child Adolesc Psychiatry 2008;17(2):63–72.
70. Berggren S, Engström AC, Bölte S. Facial affect recognition in autism, ADHD and typical development. Cogn Neuropsychiatry 2016;21(3):213–27.
71. Rao PA, Landa RJ. Association between severity of behavioral phenotype and comorbid attention deficit hyperactivity disorder symptoms in children with autism spectrum disorders. Autism 2014;18(3):272–80.
72. Bell C, Bourke C, Colhoun H, et al. The misclassification of facial expressions in generalised social phobia. J Anxiety Disord 2011;25(2):278–83.
73. Bourke C, Douglas K, Porter R. Processing of facial emotion expression in major depression: a review. Aust N Z J Psychiatry 2010;44(8):681–96.
74. Joshi G, Petty C, Wozniak J, et al. The heavy burden of psychiatric comorbidity in youth with autism spectrum disorders: a large comparative study of a psychiatrically referred population. J Autism Dev Disord 2010;40(11):1361–70.
75. Schoth DE, Liossi C. A systematic review of experimental paradigms for exploring biased interpretation of ambiguous information with emotional and neutral associations. Front Psychol 2017;8. https://doi.org/10.3389/fpsyg.2017.00171.
76. Grynberg D, Chang B, Corneille O, et al. Alexithymia and the processing of emotional facial expressions (EFEs): systematic review, unanswered questions and further perspectives. PLoS One 2012;7(8). https://doi.org/10.1371/journal.pone.0042429.
77. Montebarocci O, Surcinelli P, Rossi N, et al. Alexithymia, verbal ability and emotion recognition. Psychiatr Q 2011;82(3):245–52.
78. Bird G, Press C, Richardson DC. The role of alexithymia in reduced eye-fixation in autism spectrum conditions. J Autism Dev Disord 2011;41(11):1556–64.
79. Cook R, Brewer R, Shah P, et al. Alexithymia, not autism, predicts poor recognition of emotional facial expressions. Psychol Sci 2013;24(5):723–32.

80. Volker MA, Lopata C, Smith DA, et al. Facial encoding of children with high-functioning autism spectrum disorders. Focus Autism Other Dev Disabl 2009; 24(4):195–204.
81. Hickman L. The importance of assessing alexithymia in psychological research. PsyPAG Quarterly 2019;111:29–32.
82. Orsmond GI, Krauss MW, Seltzer MM. Peer relationships and social and recreational activities among adolescents and adults with autism. J Autism Dev Disord 2004;34(3):245–56.

Moving?

Make sure your subscription moves with you!

To notify us of your new address, find your **Clinics Account Number** (located on your mailing label above your name), and contact customer service at:

Email: journalscustomerservice-usa@elsevier.com

800-654-2452 (subscribers in the U.S. & Canada)
314-447-8871 (subscribers outside of the U.S. & Canada)

Fax number: 314-447-8029

Elsevier Health Sciences Division
Subscription Customer Service
3251 Riverport Lane
Maryland Heights, MO 63043

*To ensure uninterrupted delivery of your subscription, please notify us at least 4 weeks in advance of move.